Graves' Disease

And

Hyperthyroidism

What You Must Know

Before They Zap Your Thyroid

With Radioactive Iodine

A Ground Breaking, Revolutionary and Comprehensive Approach

Sarfraz Zaidi, MD

Graves' Disease and Hyperthyroidism

What You Must Know Before They Zap Your Thyroid With Radioactive Iodine

Second Edition, 2014

ISBN-13: 978-1481884440
ISBN-10: 1481884441

Library of Congress Control Number: 2013900851

iComet Press

6988 Calle Dia, Camarillo, CA 93012

http://www.icometpress.com

Printed in the United States of America.

Disclaimer

The information in this book is true and complete to the best of our knowledge. This book is intended only as an informative guide for those wishing to know more about health issues. The information in this book is not intended to replace the advice of a health care provider.
The author and publisher disclaim any liability for the decisions you make based on the information contained in this book. The information provided herein should not be used during any medical emergency or for the diagnosis and treatment of any medical condition.
In no way is this book intended to replace, countermand or conflict with the advice given to by your own health care provider. The information contained in this book is general and is offered with no guarantees on the part of the author or publisher. The author and publisher disclaim all liability in connection with the use of this book. The names and identifying details of people associated with events described in this book have been changed. Any similarity to actual persons is coincidental.
Any duplication or distribution of information contained herein is strictly prohibited.

I dedicate this book to my patients,

who have been my best teachers.

CONTENTS

PART 1

PART 2

Chapter 1

Why Radioactive Iodine Is Not a Good Treatment Option for Patients With Graves' Disease

If you are diagnosed with hyperthyroidism due to Graves' disease and live in the U.S., you are likely to get the following professional advice from your endocrinologist: "I'll arrange for you to receive a pill of radioactive iodine. This will cure your Graves' disease."

"Wow, that simple," you think. You are genuinely impressed. A moment later, you may ask, "Will I need to be admitted to the hospital?"

"No, it's done as an outpatient. You simply ingest a pill and go home. That's all," your endocrinologist replies.

"Will my insurance pay for it?" you ask with concern.

"Yes. We have never encountered any insurance problems with this procedure," your endocrinologist reassures you.

If you are lucky to have a few more moments of your endocrinologists' precious time and are not overwhelmed with the diagnosis of Graves' disease, you may think to ask, "Any side-effects?"

"Well, you will likely become hypothyroid (underactive thyroid), but no big deal. We will then place you on a thyroid pill."

"For how long?" you ask.

"Ohhh! It's usually a *lifelong* treatment. Don't worry. It's a very simple treatment," your endocrinologist mumbles.

"Any other side-effects?" you bravely ask.

"No, absolutely none," your endocrinologist assures you.

That's how your visit with your endocrinologist usually ends. You trust your physician and follow his advice. In a few weeks, your symptoms of *hyperthyroidism* (overactive thyroid) subside. You start to feel human again, but a few weeks later, you feel tired, start gaining weight and feel depressed. "What happened?" You want to find an answer.

You see your physician, who quite professionally breaks the news. "Now you've become hypothyroid, as we expected. No big deal. Now I'll put you on a thyroid pill and you'll be fine."

Over the next several years, you continue to *struggle* with your weight, fatigue, muscle aches and pains, thinning of hair, depression and many other symptoms of *hypothyroidism*. For each of these symptoms, you get placed on more and more medications. If you have *good* insurance, you may also be referred to various specialists and undergo quite an extensive (and expensive) diagnostic work-up, which may discover more incidental findings, but *no* real answers. You start to wonder if these symptoms are related to your thyroid. After all, these symptoms started after you received radioactive iodine. You point it out to your physician.

"Your thyroid function is within the normal range. Therefore, your symptoms cannot be due to your thyroid condition," your physician replies in an authoritative tone.

You accept your physician's explanation. "My doctor is the thyroid expert and obviously knows what he's talking about," you think to yourself. In the meantime, you continue to suffer.

Over the years, I have seen hundreds, if not thousands, of patients with this kind of medical history. I hear a lot of patients say, "Ever since radioactive iodine, my life has never been the same, doc."

The fact is most physicians, including endocrinologists, do not know how to adequately replace thyroid hormone once a patient becomes hypothyroid after radioactive iodine treatment. Frankly, they do a *lousy* job compared to what Mother Nature does. They make it sound like losing your thyroid gland function is no big deal. In fact, it is a big deal. Here is one of the reasons why.

Most physicians, including endocrinologists, treat your radioactive iodine-induced underactive thyroid state with Levothyroxine (Synthroid, Levoxyl and Unithroid are various brand names). Levothyroxine is also called T4. Now, consider this: The thyroid gland produces two thyroid hormones, *not one*. In addition to T4, it also produces T3, which is also called Liothyronine or Triiodothyronine. Doesn't it make sense to give both of these thyroid hormones, T4 as well as T3, to a hypothyroid patient?

In fact, T3 turns out to be the main hormone that carries out thyroid functions in tissues. That's why in tissues, additional T3 is generated naturally from T4. This conversion from T4 to T3 takes place due to an important enzyme, called 5'-deiodinase. Any malfunction of deiodinase obviously disrupts the conversion from T4 to T3. Unfortunately, most physicians have been brain-washed by pharmaceutical companies with the *myth* that you just need to give T4 (Synthroid, Levoxyl or Unithroid), since it will get converted into T3. Amazingly, they do not even bother to check T3 level to see if their *presumption* is true.

The fact is that T3 in the body comes from *two* sources: direct production from the thyroid gland and conversion from T4 to T3. Hence, in a given hypothyroid patient on T4 alone, T3 level will be *suboptimal* even if T4 to T3 conversion is normal. This is because that person lacks the amount of T3 that comes directly from the thyroid gland. In addition, the enzyme deiodinase does not function optimally in many people. Subsequently, in these people, even the conversion from T4 to T3 is suboptimal.

T3 is extremely important for our metabolism as well as normal functioning of various organs in the body. There are a few *enlightened* physicians, including endocrinologists, who treat hypothyroid patients with both T4 and T3. However, even then, there are a lot of issues. The fact is that we cannot do as good of a job as Mother Nature does. So <u>DO NOT</u> lose your thyroid gland *unnecessarily*.

It Is A Myth That Radioactive Iodine Does Not Have Any Side-Effects.

1. The most common side-effect is that almost everyone who gets radioactive iodine for their Graves' disease, ends up developing <u>permanent</u> hypothyroidism (Under-active thyroid).

In Addition, There Are A Lot Of Other Side-Effects.

2. In about 20% of patients, radioactive iodine can precipitate and/or worsen Graves' eye disease, called Graves' Orbitopathy (1), which is quite troublesome and difficult to treat. Rarely, you may end up losing your eyesight.

3. In some patients, radioactive iodine can cause damage to the salivary glands, which results in dry mouth, altered sense of taste and pain in the salivary glands. These symptoms are permanent and can seriously impair your quality of life.

4. Can radioactive iodine cause cancer? It is a question that conscientious endocrinologists keep asking. After you ingest the radioactive iodine (radio-isotope I-131 to be more technical) pill, it gets concentrated in the thyroid, salivary glands, stomach and urinary bladder. Obviously, there is a *genuine* concern about cancer of these organs as well as cancer of the blood cells known as leukemia.

There are scientific reports indicating a high risk for cancer with the use of radioactive iodine. An excellent study was published in 2007 in *cancer*, the official journal of the American Cancer society. In this study, investigators from Finland followed 2793 patients for 10 years, who had received radioactive iodine treatment for their hyperthyroidism. There was clearly an increased risk of cancer, especially cancer of stomach, kidney and breast in these patients treated with radioactive iodine (2).

The nuclear disaster of Chernobyl is a great example to learn from. This nuclear disaster led to a significant *increase* of *thyroid cancer* among those who were exposed to radioactive iodine and the numbers keeps increasing with the passage of time, as radiation is known to cause long-term side-effects. Radioactive iodine (I-131) is one of the major isotopes that gets released into the atmosphere after nuclear accidents. Most physicists agree there is *no absolutely safe dose of radiation* and radiation takes a long time (up to several hundred years) to dissipate. Therefore, if you receive any radiation, such as radioactive iodine to treat your Graves' disease while you are young, it may show its long-term effects as a cancer in your older years. It is a well known fact that patients with Graves' disease are at a higher risk for thyroid cancer than the general population. Is radioactive iodine treatment playing a role?

If radioactive iodine was the *only* option to treat Graves' disease, then it might be worth the risk. However, as you will learn in later chapters, there are other options.

In addition, radioactive iodine does *not* treat the root cause of Graves' disease, which is autoimmune dysfunction. Hence, you may get rid of symptoms of hyperthyroidism, but with the passage of time, you may develop other autoimmune disorders such as Celiac Disease, Colitis, Vitamin B12 deficiency, Lupus or Type 1 Diabetes.

In my early days as an endocrinologist, I used to treat Graves' disease with radioactive iodine, just like most other endocrinologists in the U.S. Fortunately, I realized this strategy is overkill, gives rise to life-long medical issues and does not even treat the root cause of Graves' disease. Slowly, I developed a comprehensive, scientific yet practical strategy, which is *free* of the influence of the pharmaceutical industry as well as *free* of the unsubstantiated *claims* of *Alternative* medicine, which often takes advantage of those who are genuinely skeptical of traditional medicine.

My strategy gets down to the root cause of Graves' disease and *uproots* it right from there. In this book, I share this strategy with you.

References:

1. Ponto KA, Zang S, Kahaly GJ. The tale of radioiodine and Graves' orbitopathy. *Thyroid.* 2010 Jul;20(7):785-93

2. Metso S, Auvinen A, Huhtala H, Salmi J, Oksala H, Jaatinen P. Increased cancer incidence after radioiodine treatment for hyperthyroidism. *Cancer.* 2007 May 15;109(10):1972-9.

Chapter 2

What is the Thyroid?

The Thyroid is an *endocrine* gland. What is an endocrine gland? An endocrine gland is a ductless gland, as compared to a gland with a duct, such as a salivary gland. For instance, a salivary gland delivers its secretion, saliva, through its duct to a local area: in this case, the oral cavity. Glands with ducts are called *exocrine* glands. As compared to an exocrine gland, an endocrine gland secretes its hormone directly into blood circulation, which then exerts its affects on distant organs in the body.

Location

The Thyroid is present in your anterior neck, lying just below the Adam's apple (thyroid cartilage), in front of the trachea (windpipe). It moves up with the act of swallowing. If enlarged, you can see it move up with swallowing. That's why your doctor asks you to swallow while inspecting and palpating your thyroid gland.

Structure

The Thyroid gland is shaped like a butterfly. It has two lobes, right and left, with a midline bridge called the isthmus.

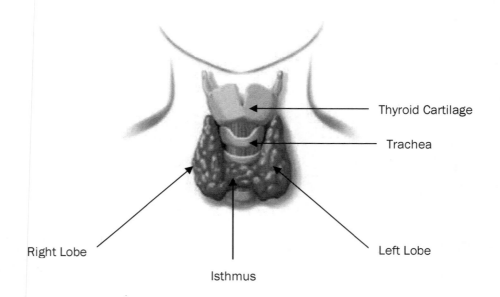

Thyroid Cartilage

Trachea

Right Lobe

Left Lobe

Isthmus

Thyroid

At the microscopic level, the thyroid gland consists of closely packed sacs called follicles. Each follicle is filled with a protein material called colloid. The wall of each follicle is comprised of a single layer of epithelial cells, called follicular cells. These are the cells that produce colloid as well as the thyroid hormones, T4 and T3. T4 is also known as Thyroxine and T3 is also known as Triiodothyronine.

Scattered in between the follicles is another kind of cell called parafollicular cells or C-cells. These cells produce a hormone called Calcitonin, which is involved in the regulation of calcium level in the blood.

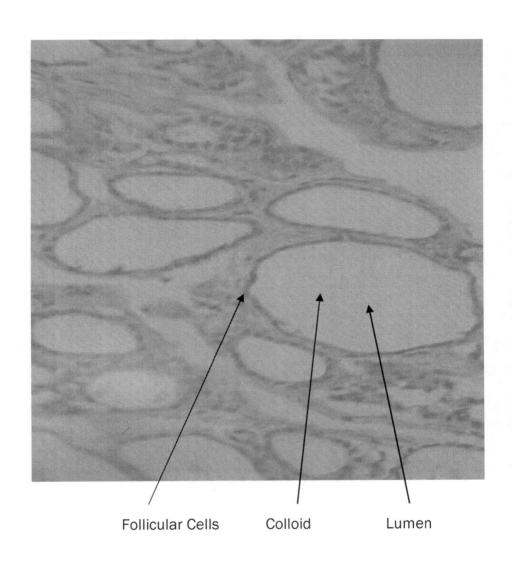

Follicular Cells   Colloid   Lumen

<u>Thyroid Follicles</u>

Function

The primary function of the thyroid gland is to produce two thyroid hormones, T4 and T3. The thyroid follicle is the basic functioning unit of the thyroid gland. Think of a follicle as a sac, lined by a layer of thyroid cells. These are called follicular cells. These cells produce a special protein called Thyroglobulin, which is then stored in the central cavity of each follicle. Synthesis of thyroid hormones takes place on this preformed thyroglobulin.

Synthesis of Thyroid Hormones

Synthesis of thyroid hormones consists of three steps:

1. Iodide Uptake

To synthesize thyroid hormones, thyroid cells need iodine, which primarily comes from diet. Iodine is a trace element which is present in variable amounts in the earth's crust. However, sea water contains fairly good amounts of iodine. Dietary iodine is converted to inorganic iodide inside the body.

Each thyroid cell has an outer (basal) wall, an inner (apical) wall and two sidewalls. The basal wall actively transports iodide from blood circulation into the cell. This is called **Iodide Uptake**. Iodide is then transported inside the thyroid cell towards its inner apical wall, where synthesis of T4 and T3 takes place.

2. Iodination

In order to produce thyroid hormones, the thyroid cell combines iodide with tyrosine, an essential amino acid present inside the thyroglobulin molecule. This process is called **iodination** of tyrosine. This chemical reaction is catalyzed by an enzyme called TPO (Thyroid Peroxidase) as well as H_2O_2 (Hydrogen Peroxide.)

As a result of iodination, two compounds are formed: MIT (Monoiodotyrosine) and DIT (Diiodotyrosine). Each MIT molecule contains one iodide atom and each DIT molecule contains two iodide atoms, attached to tyrosine.

3. Coupling

The next step, called **coupling**, occurs when two DIT molecules fuse to form a molecule that contains four iodide atoms. This is called tetraiodothyronine or thyroxine or T4. Also, one MIT fuses with one DIT, which forms a molecule that contains three iodide atoms. This is called Triiodothyronine or T3. Only T4 and T3 are *true* thyroid hormones. MIT and DIT do not possess any hormonal activity.

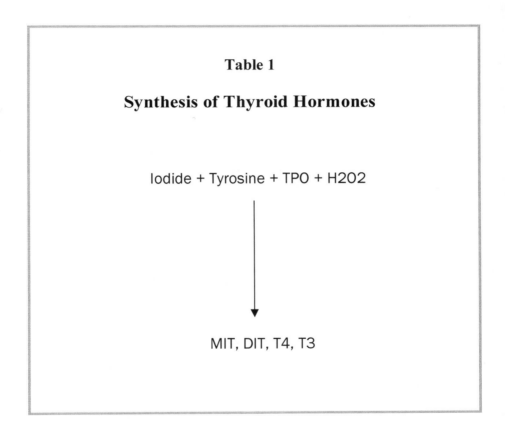

Table 1

Synthesis of Thyroid Hormones

Iodide + Tyrosine + TPO + H2O2

MIT, DIT, T4, T3

Storage

After synthesis, MIT, DIT, T3 and T4 get stored in the thyroglobulin inside the lumen of the follicle. In this way, thyroid gland serves as a large *reservoir* for storing the thyroid hormones. A normal thyroid gland stores about **8000** microgram of iodine, 90% of which is in the form of MIT, DIT, T3 and T4. Remaining 10% is in the form of iodide.

This unique storage function of the thyroid gland provides a safety-net against depletion of thyroid hormones, should synthesis ceases for some reason.

Release of T4 and T3

Small quantities of T3 and T4 are then released into blood circulation according to your body's needs. This process involves reabsorption of thyroglobulin from the follicular lumen back into the thyroid cell, where thyroglobulin undergoes breakdown. Consequently, T4, T3, DIT and MIT are freed from the thyroglobulin molecule. T3 and T4 are released into blood circulation at the basal wall of the cell. MIT and DIT remain inside the cell and undergo further breakdown, as a result of which *iodide* is freed from tyrosine. A variable amount of freed iodide gets released into blood circulation. The remaining freed iodide stays inside the cell and is recycled for reformation of MIT and DIT.

Under normal circumstances, the thyroid gland releases about **80 - 90** micrograms of T4 and **6 - 8** micrograms of T3 per day.

Transport Of T4 and T3

Most of the T4 and T3 circulate in the blood, tightly bound to proteins, the most important of which is called TBG (Thyroid Binding Globulin). The other two less important binding proteins are TBPA (Thyroid Binding PreAlbumin) and albumin.

T4 and T3 in the bound form are metabolically inactive. Only a tiny fraction, 0.03% of total T4 and 0.3% of total T3, is present as Free T4 and Free T3 respectively. It is these free fractions that are *available* to tissues. Remember, even Free T4 is metabolically *not* very active. It needs to be converted to Free T3, which is the active thyroid hormone.

T4 to T3 Conversion in the Tissues

T3 is the active thyroid hormone, responsible for all of the biological actions of the thyroid hormone. Daily total production of T3 is about **32** micrograms (mcg), about 75-80% (24-26 mcg) of which comes from T4 to T3 conversion in the peripheral tissues. However, about 20-25% (6-8 micrograms) of the total daily production of T3 comes directly from the thyroid gland.

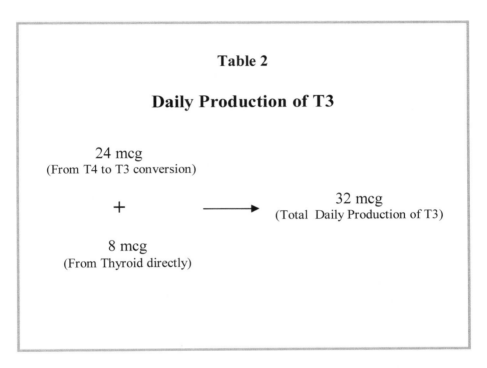

Table 2

Daily Production of T3

24 mcg
(From T4 to T3 conversion)

+   32 mcg
(Total Daily Production of T3)

8 mcg
(From Thyroid directly)

T4 to T3 conversion takes place under the guidance of an enzyme called 5'-deiodinase (DI). There are two types of 5'-DI: Type 1-DI and Type 2-DI. Type 1-DI is most abundant in the peripheral tissues, especially in the thyroid, liver, kidneys and muscles. Type 2-DI is mostly found in the brain and pituitary gland.

T4 Conversion to Inactive Reverse T3

T4 is also converted into an *inactive* form of T3 which is called reverse T3 (rT3). This conversion takes place under the guidance of another enzyme, called 5-deiodinase or Type 3 DI. Daily production of rT3 is about **19** micrograms

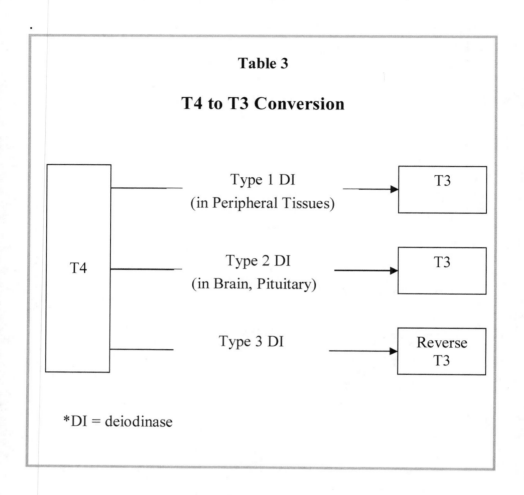

Table 3

T4 to T3 Conversion

Type 1 DI
(in Peripheral Tissues) → T3

Type 2 DI
(in Brain, Pituitary) → T3

Type 3 DI → Reverse T3

T4

*DI = deiodinase

Degradation Of T4 to other Inactive Compounds

About 70% of circulating Free T4 is converted to Free T3 and rT3 in a ratio of about 60% T3 to 40% rT3. The remaining 30% of Free T4 is converted into *Inactive* compounds through mechanisms independent of deiodinases. These mechanisms are sulfation, glucuronidation, deamination and decarboxylation of T4, primarily in the liver. These are called the *alternative* pathways of T4 degradation.

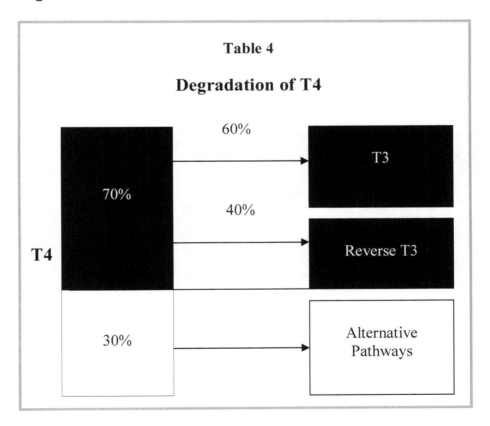

Table 4

Degradation of T4

T3 is the Active Thyroid Hormone

Out of all of the thyroid hormones, T3 is the *most* active hormone. In order to carry out the thyroid hormone function, T3 combines with Thyroid Hormone Receptor (THR) located inside the nucleus of a cell. T3 exerts its effects on almost every organ in the body, in particular the heart, brain, muscles, bones, skin, intestines and reproductive organs.

Regulation

The function of the thyroid gland is regulated in several ways:

1. The Pituitary Gland regulates thyroid hormone production by producing TSH (Thyroid Stimulating Hormone). The Pituitary Gland senses the level of T3, judges it to be normal, low or high and produces the amount of TSH in an *inverse* manner. In this way, the pituitary produces more TSH if T3 is low, and less TSH if T3 is high. TSH goes to the thyroid gland and tries to increase or decrease the production of thyroid hormones: high TSH increases and low TSH decreases the production of thyroid hormones.

2. The function of the pituitary gland is regulated by another endocrine gland, called **the hypothalamus,** which is located above the pituitary gland. The hypothalamus regulates the function of the pituitary gland by producing a number of hormones. In terms of thyroid regulation, it produces a hormone called TRH (Thyrotropin Releasing Hormone), which fine-tunes the production of TSH, which in turn regulates the production of thyroid hormones by the thyroid gland.

The hypothalamus itself is influenced by the *limbic* system, as well as various chemicals (neurotransmitters) in the brain. Limbic system is the center of our emotions. In this way, stress as well as psychiatric illnesses and medications can affect the production of your thyroid hormones, by influencing your hypothalamus and pituitary gland.

3. The Thyroid also has an incredible **auto-regulation.** For example, if there is an acute load of a *large* amount of iodine/iodide, the thyroid gland gets *saturated* with the amount of iodine it needs. Subsequently, there is a decrease in the amount of further uptake of iodine/iodide for a few days, after which uptake of iodine resumes normally. An *analogy* would be an unexpected large supply of raw material to a factory, which uses all of the raw material it can, to manufacture its product. At the same, it also reduces the demand of new raw material. A large dose of iodine/iodide also decreases the release of thyroid hormones into the circulation, temporarily.

These are primarily *protective* mechanisms against the production and release of excessive thyroid hormones in case there is a sudden supply of large quantities of the raw material, iodine/iodide. For example, contrast agents used during CT scans and angiograms contain huge quantities of iodine. In the same way, cough syrups usually contain large quantities of iodine. Iodine is also used as an antiseptic for skin cuts and wounds. Thanks to the auto-regulatory mechanisms, the vast *majority* of people do not become hyperthyroid or hypothyroid after a large load of iodine.

However, hypothyroidism or hyperthyroidism may develop *rarely*, due to the chronic use of iodine in large doses. For example, if a patient with Graves' disease continues to consume large quantities of iodine, they may develop hyperthyroidism or their pre-existing hyperthyroidism may worsen. The large quantities of iodine provide increased amounts of the raw material to the factory of the thyroid gland, which is already overactive. This is like adding fuel to the fire. Medically speaking, this phenomenon is called *Jod-Basedow's* effect.

Chapter **3**

What is Graves' Disease?

Graves' disease is named after an eminent, nineteenth century Irish surgeon, Robert James Graves, who first described the association of eye disease with an enlarged thyroid gland.

Now we know that Graves' disease is an *autoimmune* disease. It usually has a *genetic* predisposition. A family history of Graves' disease or some other autoimmune disease is usually present. Graves' disease affects females much more commonly than males, with a ratio of about 6:1. It usually starts in young age, but can happen at any age. Onset is usually insidious, but rarely it can be rather acute.

Graves' disease affects the thyroid gland in about 90% of cases, eyes in about 25-50% of cases and skin in about 1-4 % of cases.

When Graves' disease affects the thyroid gland, it causes an overproduction of thyroid hormones, which is medically called hyperthyroidism. Graves' disease usually causes diffuse enlargement of the thyroid gland, medically known as a goiter.

When Graves' disease affects the eyes, it causes what is medically known as Graves' orbitopathy or ophthalmopathy.

When Graves' Disease affects the skin, we call it Graves' dermopathy or pretibial myxedema.

Chapter **4**

Symptoms of Graves' Disease

The symptoms of Graves' Disease are usually due to an overactive thyroid, which is medically known as hyperthyroidism.

Common symptoms and signs due to hyperthyroidism are:

- Weight loss despite eating a lot
- Tremors/Shakiness
- Anxiety/Insomnia
- Irritability/Agitation
- Palpitations (rapid heart beat). Sometimes, irregular rapid heart beat, known as atrial fibrillation
- Feeling hot all the time when other people feel comfortable
- Excessive perspiration
- Diffuse enlargement of the thyroid gland, called diffuse goiter
- Too much energy followed by exhaustion
- Shortness of breath
- High blood pressure, especially systolic blood pressure
- Chest pain
- Muscle weakness
- Diarrhea
- Weakening of bone strength, known as osteopenia or osteoporosis
- High calcium in the blood
- In women, hyperthyroidism can also lead to less frequent, scanty menses and sometimes, even complete lack of menses.

- In men, hyperthyroidism can cause enlargement of breast tissue, medically known as gynecomastia.

Thyroid Storm

Rarely, patients can develop *extreme* hyperthyroidism known as Thyroid Storm. Symptoms include high grade fever, markedly increased sweating, high blood pressure, chest pain, congestive heart failure, palpitations, weakness, disorientation, irritability, confusion and psychosis.

<u>Causes of Thyroid Storm</u>

- Radioactive iodine for overactive thyroid
- Untreated hyperthyroidism for a long time
- Stress, including trauma and infections such as pneumonia
- Heart attack
- Thyroid Surgery for overactive thyroid
- Sudden stopping of anti-thyroid drugs
- Too much thyroid hormone for thyroid hormone replacement

Thyroid storm is a medical emergency and should be treated by an experienced endocrinologist.

Apathetic Hyperthyroidism in the Elderly

In the elderly, the symptoms of hyperthyroidism are few and less dramatic than what is seen in young individuals. Instead of a hyperkinetic state, there is apathy. That's why it's called <u>apathetic</u> hyperthyroidism. It was first described in medical literature by Dr. Lahey in 1931.

The usual symptoms of apathetic hyperthyroidism are depression, weakness and decreased appetite instead of high energy, agitation and increased appetite typically seen in young individuals. Chronic diarrhea and atrial fibrillation are other manifestations of apathetic hyperthyroidism in the elderly. Eye symptoms of Graves' disease are usually absent.

The diagnosis of apathetic hyperthyroidism in the elderly is often missed because a family physician typically does *not* think beyond the usual mindset of a symptom-related approach. In this case, usually the physician may think of cancer, heart disease and endogenous depression, especially if you live in the USA. Often, a patient sees a lot of specialists such as a psychiatrist, oncologist, cardiologist and gastroenterologist. Typically, a number of invasive and expensive tests are done, especially if you have good insurance. What often is *not* done is a simple blood test for thyroid and a referral to an endocrinologist. In this way, a lot of precious time gets wasted and the patient suffers unnecessarily. Sad but true!

You cannot entirely blame the family physician or other specialists who simply practice what they were trained to do. In addition, they practice *defensive* medicine to protect themselves against medical lawsuits in the USA. Undiagnosed heart disease and cancer are the two most common causes for medical lawsuits in the USA.

Graves' Orbitopathy or Ophthalmopathy

When Graves' disease affects the eyes, it is called Graves' orbitopathy or ophthalmopathy.

Symptoms include bulging of eyes, which is medically called proptosis or exophthalmos. Usually, bulging of eyes occurs in both eyes symmetrically. Sometimes, the bulging may be more pronounced on one side than the other, in which case you should have an ultrasound, CT scan or MRI scan of the orbits to exclude any tumor behind the eye.

Often, there is a feeling of irritation, a feeling of a foreign body and excessive tearing. There may be redness of the eyes due to conjunctivitis, as well as blurry vision and sensitivity to light due to corneal ulceration. Some patients may feel pressure behind the eyes. Occasionally, there may be severe pain, which is an emergency for which you should call your physician immediately or go to the Emergency Room at a hospital.

Sometimes, you may start to see double, usually in the upward gaze, but double vision can be in any direction. Initially, double vision is intermittent, but later it can be present all the time. Rarely, Graves' orbitopathy can lead to decreased vision and even blindness if left untreated.

Symptoms of eye disease usually develop *concurrently* with symptoms of hyperthyroidism. However, eye disease may *precede* or develop *after* the symptoms of hyperthyroidism.

Graves' Dermopathy/Pretibial Myxedema

Rarely, patients with Graves' disease may also experience a peculiar thickening of skin on the shins. It is best described as an orange peel. This is known as Graves' dermopathy or pretibial myxedema.

Asymptomatic Graves' Disease

Rarely, patients with Graves' disease do not have any symptoms. They get diagnosed with Graves' disease because their physician does a battery of laboratory tests including thyroid antibodies. I like to consider this condition an early stage of Graves' disease. This does not require any drug treatment, radioactive iodine or surgery. However, it does require treatment of the underlying autoimmune disorder, as is outlined later in this book.

Chapter **5**

Diagnosis of Graves' Disease

In most cases, the diagnosis of Graves' disease is *pretty* obvious. Unfortunately, it is often *missed* for some time, as physicians generally *chase* individual symptoms by doing extensive imaging testing and referring to various specialists, except for an endocrinologist.

Often, patients come to see me after they have been to a cardiologist for their palpitations, a gynecologist for their heat intolerance, a psychiatrist for their anxiety and agitation, a rheumatologist for their muscle weakness and an ophthalmologist for their eye symptoms. One of the physicians along the way decides to do a blood test for thyroid function, which usually confirms that the patient has hyperthyroidism.

The blood test for thyroid function is comprised of: TSH (Thyroid Stimulating Hormone), Free T3 and Free T4.

In hyperthyroidism, TSH is typically below the normal range and often suppressed, while Free T3 and Free T4 are generally elevated. However, in mild cases of hyperthyroidism, Free T3 and Free T4 may be in the normal range, but only TSH is below the normal range. In medical terms, we call it Subclinical Hyperthyroidism.

Once the diagnosis of hyperthyroidism is confirmed, the next step is to find out the *cause* of hyperthyroidism, Graves' disease being one of them.

Causes of Hyperthyroidism

- Graves' disease
- Too large a dose of thyroid hormone in patients with underactive thyroid
- Surreptitious use of thyroid hormone, often to lose weight or have more energy
- Subacute Thyroiditis
- Post-partum (post-delivery) Thyroiditis
- Painless Thyroiditis
- Drugs such as amiodarone, interferon
- Toxic multinodular goiter
- Hyperemesis Gravidarum during Pregnancy, Molar pregnancy (a rare cause), Ovarian Tumor (a rare cause)
- TSH producing pituitary tumor (extremely rare)

One has to sort out between these various causes of hyperthyroidism. This is where an endocrinologist is indispensible. An experienced endocrinologist puts all of the clinical features of a patient into perspective and can readily make a clinical diagnosis of Graves' disease in most instances.

Thyroid Antibodies Tests

Often, the endocrinologist orders a blood test for thyroid antibodies to confirm his/her clinical impression. This test typically is to check for thyroid antibodies.

Four thyroid antibody tests:

- Anti-TPO (Thyroid PerOxidase) antibody.
- Anti-Tg (ThyroGlobulin) antibody.
- Thyroid Stimulating Immunoglobulin (TSI).
- Thyrotropin Receptor Antibody (TRAB).

Blood tests for anti-TPO and anti-Tg antibodies are easily available, cheap and the most commonly used thyroid antibody tests. If these antibodies are elevated, it indicates autoimmune thyroid disease. In the right clinical setting, these two antibody tests are sufficient to confirm the diagnosis of Graves' disease.

Blood test for TSI is the most specific test for Graves' disease. TRAB is also used to diagnose Graves' disease, but is less specific than TSI. Both of these tests are more expensive, less commonly done and may not be readily available. I use these tests only rarely. In my clinical practice, I routinely diagnose Graves' disease clinically and simply order tests for anti-TPO and anti-Tg antibodies to confirm the diagnosis. Only rarely do I order TSI or TRAB.

Caution:

Like any other medical test, all of these antibody tests can have false positive as well as false negative results. That's why these tests, like any other test, should be interpreted in the *right* clinical settings by an *experienced* physician.

Unfortunately, these days many physicians in the USA order a lot of *unnecessary* tests due to medico-legal concerns as well as pressure from patients to find any *possible* medical problem. Then, these physicians *chase* the so-called *abnormal* test with a number of more expensive tests which usually leads to referrals to a number of specialists, each one ordering more tests and in the end, giving vague answers to the patient. This kind of medical practice not only incurs *huge* medical bills, but also causes a lot of *stress* for patients as well as physicians.

Radioiodine Uptake and Scan of Thyroid

Rarely, the endocrinologist will resort to a special test called radioiodine uptake and scan of thyroid, especially in order to differentiate Graves' hyperthyroidism from Subacute thyroiditis and Painless thyroiditis. Thyroid radioiodine uptakes are typically *high* in Graves' hyperthyroidism, but very *low* in Subacute thyroiditis and Painless thyroiditis.

Caution

The results of the thyroid radioiodine uptake and scan should be interpreted by an endocrinologist in the context of the overall clinical picture of the patient. Sometimes, an overzealous radiologist may over-interpret the test, which can lead to misdiagnosis if an endocrinologist is not involved in the care of the patient. For example, a radiologist may suggest that the patient has hypothyroidism (Underactive Thyroid), based upon low uptake values of radioiodine, which are not only seen in hypothyroidism, but also typically seen in cases of hyperthyroidism (overactive thyroid) due to Subacute thyroiditis, Post-partum thyroiditis as well as Painless thyroiditis. A family physician (typically in the HMO setting) may follow the radiologist's advice and put this patient on thyroid hormone replacement, which is like *adding fuel to the fire*. Then, the patient may end up with a *serious* medical emergency. I have actually encountered these kinds of *messed* up cases.

Chapter **6**

Other Causes of Hyperthyroidism

Graves' disease is *not* the only cause of hyperthyroidism (overactive thyroid).

Besides Graves' disease, here is a list of various conditions that can cause hyperthyroidism.

- Too large a dose of thyroid hormone in patients with underactive thyroid
- Surreptitious use of thyroid hormone, often to lose weight or have more energy
- Subacute Thyroiditis
- Post-partum (post-delivery) Thyroiditis
- Painless Thyroiditis
- Drugs such as amiodarone, interferon
- Toxic nodular goiter
- Hyperemesis Gravidarum during Pregnancy, Molar pregnancy (a rare cause), Ovarian Tumor (a rare cause)
- TSH producing pituitary tumor (extremely rare)

Subacute Thyroiditis

Subacute thyroiditis refers to inflammation of the thyroid gland, which has a clinical course of several weeks. Usually it is triggered by an acute upper respiratory tract infection (URI), such as a common cold.

Symptoms occur in two phases:

Symptoms of hyperthyroidism:

- Pain in the thyroid area. At times, pain also radiates to the ear.
- Restlessness
- Palpitations
- Insomnia/anxiety
- Excessive perspiration
- Intolerance to heat
- Excessive weight loss despite good appetite

A few (6-12) weeks later, these symptoms subside on their own and symptoms of hypothyroidism develop, which typically include:

- Fatigue, sluggishness
- Weight gain
- Intolerance to cold
- Depressed mood

What Causes Subacute Thyroiditis?

The cause of subacute thyroiditis is an inflammation of the thyroid gland, secondary to an upper respiratory tract infection (URI), which causes structural damage to the thyroid gland. It's like a tornado hitting a trailer park.

Normally, the thyroid gland stores a large amount of thyroid hormones to be released in small quantities over a period of time.

With the destruction of the gland caused by the tornado of subacute thyroiditis, the large quantities of the stored thyroid hormones gets released into the blood circulation. This causes the phase of hyperthyroidism.

The thyroid hormones remain in circulation for a few weeks (6-12 weeks) and so does the phase of hyperthyroidism.

After the tornado goes away, the thyroid gland starts to repair itself, but it takes a while.

During this period, there is shortage of thyroid hormones, which gives rise to the phase of hypothyroidism. This phase typically last a few weeks (6-12 weeks).

Eventually, in most cases, the thyroid gland restores back to normal, although some patients may become hypothyroid permanently.

Diagnosis of Subacute Thyroiditis

Diagnosis of subacute thyroiditis is a tricky one. Patients usually consult their family physicians, who often do not think about the possibility of subacute thyroiditis. Patients get placed on a variety of medicines to control their symptoms which do not get better and they feel quite frustrated. Usually, it takes an endocrinologist to diagnose subacute thyroiditis.

Diagnostic Tests include:

- TSH, Free T4, FreeT3
- Thyroid Antibody tests
- Thyroid Radioiodine uptake and scan

Thyroid Radioiodine uptake and scan is the *most* useful tool in deciding whether hyperthyroidism is due to subacute thyroiditis or Graves' disease. In subacute thyroiditis, radioiodine uptake is minimal. On the other hand, it is elevated in Graves' disease.

The Thyroid Radioiodine uptake and scan should **not** be done if a patient is pregnant or breast-feeding.

Treatment of Subacute Thyroiditis

In the majority of cases, subacute thyroiditis is a self-limiting disease. Therefore, no specific treatment is required. However, close monitoring is essential.

Symptoms of hyperthyroidism can be managed with a Beta-Blocker such as atenolol or propranolol.

If pain in the thyroid area is intolerable, a short course of oral steroids, such as Prednisone, is quite helpful.

Symptoms of hypothyroidism may require a short course of thyroid hormone replacement with T4 and T3.

Patient education and close monitoring of the thyroid functions are the most important component of the treatment.

Painless Thyroiditis/Silent Thyroiditis

Painless thyroiditis refers to a condition of inflammation of the thyroid gland. However, as compared to subacute thyroiditis, which causes a lot of pain in the neck, painless thyroiditis is painless. It is also called Silent Thyroiditis.

Its clinical course, diagnosis and treatment is similar to that of subacute Thyroiditis.

Postpartum Thyroiditis

Postpartum thyroiditis refers to thyroiditis that develops in women after they have delivered a baby.

Its clinical course, diagnosis and treatment is similar to that of subacute Thyroiditis.

Diagnosis of postpartum thyroiditis is a tricky one. Patients usually consult their obstetrician or family physicians who often do not think about the possibility of postpartum thyroiditis. They blame symptoms of hyperthyroidism on anxiety of motherhood and symptoms of hypothyroidism on postpartum depression.

Patients get placed on a variety of medicines to control their symptoms which do not get better and they feel quite frustrated.

Caution:

The radio-iodine uptake and scan should **NOT** be done if a patient is breast-feeding because of the risk of transmitting radiation to the baby through milk. In that case, clinical monitoring is usually the best option, as hyperthyroidism due to postpartum thyroiditis usually resolves in 6-12 weeks, but does not resolve in the case of Graves' disease.

If it is important to get a diagnosis on an urgent basis, then either the mother can decide to stop breast feeding or pump and store her breast milk in a refrigerator for about 5-7 days supply. By that time, it is safe to resume breast feeding.

Drug-Induced Hyperthyroidism

Occasionally, drugs can give rise to hyperthyroidism. Amiodarone is the most notorious drug in this regard. This is a drug to treat heart arrhythmias.

Sometimes, interferon can also cause hyperthyroidism. It is important to remember the possible connection between these drugs and symptoms of hyperthyroidism. You need to consult an experienced endocrinologist for proper evaluation and treatment.

Toxic Nodular Goiter

A relatively common cause of hyperthyroidism is a nodular goiter. A goiter simply means an enlarged thyroid gland. A nodule is a growth within the thyroid gland, which is often benign. Rarely, it can be malignant.

In the case of a Toxic Nodular Goiter, often there are multiple nodules, which are hyper-functioning, giving rise to hyperthyroidism. Toxic simply means that the goiter is giving rise to hyperthyroidism. Rarely, there may be a single hyper-functioning nodule.

Patients with Graves' disease usually have a goiter as well, but this goiter is typically diffuse. That's why it is called Toxic Diffuse Goiter, which is another name for Graves' disease.

In case of a Toxic Nodular Goiter, usually a person has a visible goiter for a number of years with normal thyroid function. Then, hyperthyroidism develops very slowly. This is in sharp contrast to Graves' disease, where hyperthyroidism develops rapidly and the goiter is diffuse, not nodular. However, rarely a nodule may be present in the thyroid gland of a Graves' disease patient. It may carry a higher than normal risk of malignancy, and therefore, an ultrasound-guided Fine Needle Aspiration (FNA) biopsy should be considered in a Graves' disease patient with a thyroid nodule.

Symptoms of hyperthyroidism in a toxic nodular goiter are usually minimal. In the elderly, the only symptoms may be new onset atrial fibrillation or congestive heart failure. Rarely, a multi-nodular goiter may cause some pressure symptoms, such as compression on the trachea, difficulty swallowing or hoarseness of voice.

Diagnosis is based on the clinical findings of a nodular goiter and a low TSH. Free T3 and Free T4 may be normal or elevated.

The next step is to do a Radioiodine uptake and scan to confirm the hyper-functioning status of these nodules, which manifest as hot nodules on the scan. What is a hot nodule? When a nodule takes up more radioiodine than usual uptake by the rest of the gland, it is called a hot nodule. Hot nodules are almost never malignant.

An Ultrasound of the thyroid should also be done to evaluate the size and other features of the nodules. Usually, a multi-nodular gland with hyperthyroidism is non-malignant. However, if there is a large nodule, or if a nodule starts to enlarge or has suspicious features on an ultrasound, an ultrasound-guided Fine Needle Aspiration (FNA) biopsy should be considered to exclude malignancy.

Treatment of Toxic nodular goiter is with surgery. Occasionally, radioactive iodine is employed in an elderly patient, whose overall health may be too poor to undergo surgery.

Chapter 7

Traditional Treatment

of Graves' Disease

In the traditional, customary medical approach, three options are available to treat hyperthyroidism due to Graves' disease.

- Anti-thyroid drugs
- Radioactive Iodine (I-131)
- Surgery

Let's take a close look at each one of these options.

1. Anti-thyroid Drugs

There are three anti-thyroid drugs available around the world. All are available in pill form.

- **Methimazole (MMI)**
- **Propylthiouracil (PTU)**
- **Carbimazole**

In the U.S., only two drugs are available: Methimazole (brand name Tapazole) and Propylthiouracil or PTU. In many parts of the world, Carbimazole is often used to treat Graves' disease. Carbimazole gets converted into Methimazole in the body.

How Do Anti-Thyroid Drugs Work?

Anti-thyroid drugs work by blocking the synthesis of thyroid hormone in the Thyroid gland. Compared to radioactive iodine, these drugs do not cause permanent damage to the thyroid gland. Typically, you take an anti-thyroid drug for a period of about 18-24 months and then stop it. In general, you have a 50% chance that your hyperthyroidism will be cured, but you also have a 50% chance that hyperthyroidism will recur once you stop the anti-thyroid drug.

Methimazole has a half life of about 4-6 hours. Therefore, it needs to be taken only once or twice a day. In comparison, PTU has a shorter half life of about 75 minutes. Therefore, it needs to be taken three times or sometimes even four times a day.

For the convenience of dosing, Methimazole is usually the preferred drug. However, PTU is the preferred drug during pregnancy as Methimazole can rarely cause a serious skin disorder in the fetus. This defect in the skin of a newborn is called cutis aplasia. It is often small and usually localized to the scalp, but it can be anywhere on the body and can occur as multiple skin defects.

Side-Effects of Anti-thyroid Drugs

Anti-thyroid drugs are old drugs. Propylthiouracil and Methimazole were approved in 1947 and 1950, respectively (1).

These are generally well tolerated, but rarely side-effects may develop. These side-effects can be *minor* such as itching, skin rash, joint pains, migraine headaches and stomach upset. *Major side effects include* liver toxicity, vasculitis (inflammation of blood vessels) and granulocytopenia (a decrease in the number of white blood cells). Granulocytopenia is usually transient, but in some cases, it can progress to suppression of bone marrow, termed agranulocytosis, which is a serious medical condition and can be fatal.

Liver toxicity and vasculitis are more common with PTU (Propylthiouracil) than with Methimazole. Liver toxicity occurs rarely, in about 0.1 % of cases. In 2009, the FDA issued an alert regarding PTU-induced liver injury. Its Adverse Event Reporting System (AERS) has identified 32 cases of serious liver injury associated with the use of PTU over the past 20 years. Among them, 22 were adults and 10 were children. Among these adults, 12 deaths and 5 liver transplants took place. Among children, 1 death and 6 liver transplants occurred.

In contrast, 5 cases of serious liver injury were identified with the use of Methimazole. All five cases were in adult patients and 3 resulted in death (1).

PTU treatment during pregnancy resulted in two cases of serious maternal liver injury and there were two cases of liver injury in fetuses whose mothers took PTU (2).

The average daily dose of PTU associated with liver failure was approximately 300 mg in both children and adults. Liver failure occurred after 6 to 450 days (median, 120 days) of treatment (2). It is estimated that each year, one or two individuals with Graves' disease in the United States will die or require a liver transplant after PTU treatment (2). The risk of PTU-related severe liver failure appears to be higher in children than in adults (2). In conclusion, PTU should be used only if a person cannot take Methimazole. This is particularly true in the case of children.

Symptoms of liver failure include fatigue, weakness, vague abdominal pain, loss of appetite, itching, easy bruising or yellowing of the eyes or skin. If you develop these symptoms, it is best to stop the anti-thyroid drug, inform your physician and have your liver function tested immediately.

Agranulocytosis occurs very rarely, in about 0.02% of cases, which translates into 2 patients out of 10,000. If the drug is stopped, full recovery may or may not take place. It usually develops early in the course of treatment, within 2 months, but can develop even later.

Granulocytopenia and agranulocytosis predisposes an individual to serious life-threatening infections and can be fatal. Therefore, these drugs should be prescribed only by endocrinologists who are experienced in using these drugs. If you develop fever or severe sore throat, it is best to stop the drug, consult your physician and have your blood tested for <u>white cell count</u>.

If you suspect your anti-thyroid drug is causing any side-effect, immediately contact your physician. It is best to stop the drug and have your blood tested for an appropriate blood test, such as <u>white cell count</u> and <u>liver function test</u>. If these tests are normal, you may want to go back on the anti-thyroid drug, after consulting your physician.

In the prestigious textbook of DeGroot's Endocrinology, J. Maxwell McKenzie and Margita Zakarija from the University of Miami describe their own experience with the side-effects of anti-thyroid drugs. In their 35 years of experience, they encountered only 1 case of agranulocytosis (3). It was induced by PTU. Full spontaneous recovery took place within 10 days after stopping the drug.

However, serious side effects of anti-thyroid drugs are low compared to the serious side effects of Radioactive Iodine as a treatment option. With the use of Radioactive iodine, there is an incidence of 0.3% of radioiodine-induced thyroid storm, which translates into <u>30 cases per 10,000 (4)</u>. Thyroid storm is a serious medical emergency and carries a high mortality of about 20%, despite aggressive medical therapy.

2. Radioactive Iodine

As discussed earlier, Radioactive Iodine is the most popular treatment option among endocrinologists in the USA. In other countries, it is used much less commonly. Instead, anti-thyroid drugs are the <u>first line</u> choice. Radioactive iodine is used if anti-thyroid drugs fail, have side-effects or have a contraindication to its use. Radioactive iodine must *not* be used in pregnant and lactating women.

How Does Radioactive Iodine Work?

Normally, your thyroid gland takes up iodine in your food to synthesize thyroid hormone. In radioactive iodine treatment, this basic principle is *exploited* to fool your thyroid gland. You ingest a pill of radioisotope of iodine, I-131 in a dose of about 9-12 mCi, which is taken up by the thyroid gland cells, but this time these cells have ingested a <u>poison</u>. The radiation emitted by I-131 kills thyroid cells permanently.

How Long Does It Take To Control Hyperthyroidism?

Often, your physician initially places you on an anti-thyroid drug to control your hyperthyroidism for a few weeks before I-131 treatment is given. It takes about four to six weeks before an anti-thyroid drug is able to bring down your thyroid hormone level in the blood. During this time, physicians often use a beta-blocking drug such as Propranolol or Atenolol to slow down your rapid heart rate, tremors and shakiness.

You stop the anti-thyroid drug for a few days (depending upon which drug is being used) prior to I-131 ingestion. I-131 does not control your hyperthyroidism immediately. It takes a few weeks (6-12 weeks) to control hyperthyroidism. During this period, you often continue to take an anti-thyroid drug.

After about 12 weeks, most people become hypothyroid (Underactive thyroid).

Then, your physician stops your anti-thyroid drug and places you on thyroid hormone replacement therapy for the **rest** of your life.

As mentioned earlier, most physicians place you on T4 alone (Levothyroxine, Synthroid, Levoxyl, Unithroid or some other brand names), without any consideration given to T3. Consequently, you continue to suffer from symptoms of hypothyroidism.

Rarely, a single dose of radioactive iodine is ineffective in controlling hyperthyroidism. Then, you need a second dose of I-131. Usually, you should wait about a <u>year</u> before deciding for the second dose of I-131.

What Are The Side-Effects Of Radioactive-Iodine?

Radioactive-iodine is quoted as being cheap and without side-effects. In fact, both of these claims are <u>false</u>. In the short term, it is cheap, but in the long-term it is very costly, because you have to take thyroid hormone pills for the rest of your life.

As discussed earlier, Radioactive iodine has a lot of side-effects.

A. Permanent Hypothyroidism

Almost everyone develops permanent hypothyroidism   after radioactive iodine treatment. This is a major side- effect. Life is never the same after you develop hypothyroidism.

B. Graves' Orbitopathy

Graves' eye disease, which is also known as Graves' orbitopathy, usually gets worse after a patient receives radioactive iodine to treat hyperthyroidism. About 20 % of patients with Graves' disease treated with radioactive iodine develop *new severe* eye disease. Symptoms of Graves' orbitopathy include bulging of eyes, irritation of eyes, "sand in the eye" feeling, excessive tearing, redness of eyes, double vision and rarely, even loss of vision.

What is the mechanism?

Radioactive iodine damages the thyroid gland and causes release of TSH-receptors into blood circulation, which provokes a severe immune reaction, causing activation of lymphocytes in your blood. Then, the activated lymphocytes can attack your eyes, as eyes contain TSH-receptors. In other words, activated lymphocytes *mistakenly* think your eyes are your thyroid gland and start to attack them.

C. Permanent Damage To Salivary Glands

Radioactive iodine can cause permanent damage to the salivary glands, symptoms of which include dry mouth, altered taste and painful swelling of the salivary glands.

D. Increased Risk For Cancer

The potential *carcinogenic* properties of radioactive iodine can increase your risk of cancer, especially in organs which take up radioactive iodine in high concentration. These organs include the thyroid, salivary glands, stomach, intestine, kidneys and urinary tract.

There are scientific reports indicating a high risk for cancer with the use of radioactive iodine. An excellent study was published in 2007 in *cancer*, the official journal of the American Cancer society. In this study, investigators from Finland followed 2793 patients for 10 years, who had received radioactive iodine treatment for their hyperthyroidism. There was clearly an increased risk of cancer, especially cancer of stomach, kidney and breast in these patients treated with radioactive iodine (5).

E. Worsening Of Hyperthyroidism

In some patients, radioactive iodine can cause acute inflammation of the thyroid gland, known as *radiation thyroiditis*. In these cases, there is a sudden release of a large amount of the preformed thyroid hormone, which is normally stored in the thyroid gland, into blood circulation.

Consequently, there is an acute *exacerbation* of the symptoms of hyperthyroidism, such as heart palpitation, tremors, anxiety, insomnia and weight loss. Rarely, it can lead to *thyroid storm*, as was mentioned earlier.

Rarely, even airway obstruction due to the swollen, inflamed thyroid gland has been reported (6).

F. Primary Hyperparathyroidism

Rarely, radioiodine treatment can cause primary hyperparathyroidism in Graves' disease patients (7). Primary hyperparathyroidism manifests as high calcium, low phosphorus and an elevated Parathyroid Hormone (PTH) level in the blood. If left untreated, it can lead to kidney stones, osteoporosis and marked elevation in blood calcium level, which can be life-threatening.

G. Acute Leukemia

Rarely, acute leukemia can develop after radioiodine treatment for Graves' disease (8).

H. Autoimmune Process Continues

Radioactive iodine treats the *symptoms* of hyperthyroidism, but does *not* treat the underlying autoimmune process. Therefore, a patient with Graves' disease who has previously received radioactive iodine is usually under the *false* impression that her Graves' disease is cured. In fact, in pregnant females, she still may have thyroid antibodies, which cross the placenta and then can cause serious thyroid disease in the newborn (9).

The autoimmune process not only causes Graves' disease, but can also lead to a number of other autoimmune diseases.

Some examples of autoimmune diseases:
- Asthma
- Eczema
- Ulcerative Colitis
- Crohns' Disease
- Irritable Bowel Syndrome
- Gluten Sensitivity/Celiac disease
- Peptic Ulcer Disease
- Vitamin B12 Deficiency
- Pernicious Anemia
- Type 1 Diabetes
- Adrenal Insufficiency/Addison's disease
- Multiple Sclerosis (M.S.)
- Chronic rheumatologic conditions (such as Rheumatoid Arthritis, Fibromyalgia, Systemic Lupus Erythematosis, commonly known as Lupus and Ankylosing Spondylitis).

3. Surgery

Surgery is rarely done in Graves' disease patients, because of the following reasons:

A. Risk Of Anesthesia

Why put patients under the risk of anesthesia when Graves' disease can be effectively treated with anti-thyroid drugs or radioactive iodine?

B. Low Calcium In The Blood

In addition to anesthesia, there are known complications of thyroid surgery, which include <u>low calcium</u> in the blood due to Hypoparathyroidism (low level of Parathyroid hormone), which can be life-threatening.

Often, it is transient, but can be permanent in some cases. Hypoparathyroidism develops as a result of injury to the four parathyroid glands, which are embedded in the thyroid gland. This injury may be transient or permanent.

C. Hoarseness Of Voice

Other complications of thyroid surgery include injury to the recurrent laryngeal nerve, which results in hoarseness of voice. It can be permanent.

D. Permanent Hypothyroidism

Permanent hypothyroidism is often a late complication of subtotal thyroid resection, known as Subtotal Thyroidectomy. However, in the case of total thyroid resection, known as Total Thyroidectomy, hypothyroidism results soon after surgery.

E. Worsening Of Graves' Eye Disease

Eyes disease due to Graves' disease can be worsened after thyroid surgery.

F. Expensive

Surgery is much more expensive than anti-thyroid drugs or radioactive iodine.

G. Autoimmune Process Continues

Like radioactive iodine, surgery also does *not* treat the underlying root cause of Graves' disease, which is the autoimmune disease process.

Surgery is done rarely, only as a *last* resort in those occasional patients who cannot tolerate anti-thyroid drugs or radioactive iodine.

How Endocrinologists In Different Parts Of The World Treat Graves' Disease

Treatment of Graves' disease is *not* always based on science. Social, political and economic factors significantly influence the decision of physicians.

An interesting study surveyed endocrinologists in the United States, Europe and Japan in this respect (10). A majority of U.S. physicians (69%) chose radioactive iodine, compared to 22% of European physicians and only 11% of Japanese physicians. Only 30.5% of US physicians chose anti-thyroid drugs as the first-line therapy compared to 77% of Europeans and 88% of Japanese. Most endocrinologists from all three regions agreed *not* to use surgery as a first line option except in few situations.

In the U.S., physicians are very fearful of lawsuits. That's why they are afraid to use anti-thyroid drugs. They are *mistakenly* under the impression that agranulocytosis is a fairly common side-effect. As I pointed out earlier, it happens in 2 out of 10,000 cases. Outside the U.S., where physicians are not fearful of lawsuits, most physicians use anti-thyroid drugs as the first line therapy for Graves' disease.

In Conclusion

The customary treatment of Graves' disease is unsatisfactory, to say the least. What's even more disheartening is the fact that it has not changed since the 1950's.

Using radioactive iodine or surgery to treat hyperthyroidism in Graves' disease is an *unscientific, myopic* and *radical* approach. Why unscientific? Because radioactive iodine or surgery does *not* treat the underlying root cause - the autoimmune process. Hence, it is unscientific.

Why myopic? Radioactive iodine and surgery may control hyperthyroidism, but they also give rise to a number of other serious health issues, permanent hypothyroidism being a major problem. In addition, they give rise to a host of other potential complications, as we observed earlier. That's why this approach is myopic.

Why radical? Using radioactive iodine and surgery to treat a medical issue that arises out of autoimmune dysfunction, is an *overkill*. Hence, it is radical. It's like dropping a nuclear bomb on a country to kill every living thing because its leaders are not listening to us.

How about anti-thyroid drugs? The main drawback with anti-thyroid drugs is their lack of efficacy to cure hyperthyroidism: about 50% of patients have recurrence of hyperthyroidism once drugs are stopped.

Obviously, there is a need to discover a scientific, sensible and effective strategy to treat Graves' disease, something I realized soon after I became an endocrinologist.

Before we can scientifically treat Graves' disease (or any disease for that matter), we obviously need to find out what *really* causes it. Let's explore this very question in the next chapter.

References:

1.http://www.fda.gov/Drugs/DrugSafety/PostmarketDrugSafetyInfor
mationforPatientsandProviders/DrugSafetyInformationforHeathcare
Professionals/ucm162701.htm

2.http://jcem.endojournals.org/content/94/6/1881.full#ref-7

3. J. Maxwell McKenzie, Margita Zakarija. Endocrinology/edited by
Leslie DeGroot et al, Vol.1, 3rd edition. W.B. Saunders Company,
1995.

4. McDermott MT, Kidd GS, Dodson LE Jr, Hofeldt FD. Radioiodine-
induced thyroid storm. Case report and literature review. *Am J Med*.
1983 Aug;75(2):353-9.

5. Metso S, Auvinen A, Huhtala H, Salmi J, Oksala H, Jaatinen P.
Increased cancer incidence after radioiodine treatment for
hyperthyroidism. *Cancer*. 2007 May 15;109(10):1972-9.

6. Kinuya S, Yoneyama T, Michigishi T. Airway complication occurring
during radioiodine treatment for Graves' disease. *Ann Nucl Med*.
2007 Aug;21(6):367-9.

7. Colaço SM, Si M, Reiff E, Clark OH. Hyperparathyroidism after
radioactive iodine therapy. *Am J Surg*. 2007 Sep;194(3):323-7.

8. Kolade VO, Bosinski TJ, Ruffy EL. Acute promyelocytic leukemia
after iodine-131 therapy for Graves' disease. *Pharmacotherapy*.
2005 Jul;25(7):1017-20.

9. Zimmerman D. Fetal and neonatal hyperthyroidism. *Thyroid*. 1999
Jul;9(7):727-33.

10. Wartofsky L, Glinoer D, Solomon B, Nagataki S, Lagasse R,
Nagayama Y, Izumi M. Differences and similarities in the diagnosis
and treatment of Graves' disease in Europe, Japan, and the United
States. *Thyroid*. 1991;1(2):129-35.

Chapter **8**

What Really Causes Graves' Disease?

Graves' disease is an *autoimmune* disease of the thyroid gland. In this disease, your <u>immune system</u> starts to produce antibodies which are *directed* at the thyroid gland. These antibodies are *stimulatory* in nature. That's why we call them <u>Thyroid Stimulating Immunoglobulins or TSI</u>. In fact, these antibodies are directed at the TSH receptor on the thyroid cells. That's why these antibodies are also called <u>TSH receptor antibodies</u>. TSH is also called Thyrotropin. Therefore, these antibodies are also called Thyrotropin Receptor Antibodies or TRAB.

These antibodies *force* the thyroid cells to produce increased quantities of thyroid hormone. Large quantities of thyroid hormone produce signs and symptoms of hyperthyroidism (overactive thyroid).

About 25-50% of patients with Graves' disease also experience eye disease, known as Graves' orbitopathy or ophthalmopathy. Like most endocrinologists, I prefer the term Graves' orbitopathy.

In Graves' orbitopathy, the <u>immune system</u> attacks the soft tissues behind the eyeball and the extra-ocular muscles (six small muscles around each eyeball that are responsible for eye movement), which then become *inflamed* and *swollen*. This results in pushing the eyes forward, which causes bulging eyes, known as proptosis or exophthalmos. Swelling of the muscles can also compress on the venous drainage of the eyes, causing *swelling* and *inflammation* of the eyes. Swollen, inflamed muscles restrict the movement of the eyeball, which causes double vision. Severe compression of the optic nerve by inflamed tissues can threaten eyesight.

Rarely, the <u>immune system</u> attacks the subcutaneous tissues, which causes marked thickening, inflammation and swelling of the skin, giving the affected skin an *orange peel* appearance. We call it Graves' dermopathy. It usually affects the anterior lower legs. That's why it is also called pretibial myxedema. In severe cases, Graves' dermopathy can involve other parts of the body as well.

What Really Causes An Autoimmune Disease?

Because your immune system starts to attack your <u>own</u> thyroid cells, eyeball tissues or subcutaneous tissues, we call Graves' disease an auto-immune disease. But what causes an autoimmune disease? If you ask your physician, the likely response will be, "Oh, we know genetics is a factor. Besides that, we don't know much about it."

Even if you do a search on the internet or read textbooks on Graves' disease, you won't find any more useful information in this regard.

Genetics

It is true that autoimmune diseases, including Graves' Disease, tend to congregate in families. You're at a high risk of developing an autoimmune disease if you have a family history of an autoimmune disease. For example, your mother may have Hashimoto's Thyroiditis or Graves' Disease, while your sister may have Asthma or Crohns' Disease. Your brother may have Lactose Intolerance.

Here is a list of various autoimmune diseases.

- Autoimmune Thyroid Disease, which can either cause you to have a *low* level of thyroid hormone (Hashimoto's Thyroiditis) or a *high* level of thyroid hormone (Graves' Disease).
- Peptic Ulcer Disease

- Gluten Sensitivity/Celiac Disease
- Irritable Bowel Syndrome
- Ulcerative Colitis
- Crohns' Disease
- Vitamin B12 Deficiency
- Pernicious Anemia
- Type 1 Diabetes
- Adrenal Insufficiency/Addison's disease
- Asthma
- Eczema
- Psoriasis
- Multiple Sclerosis (M.S.)
- Chronic rheumatologic conditions (such as Rheumatoid Arthritis, Fibromyalgia, Systemic Lupus Erythematosis (commonly known as Lupus) and Ankylosing Spondylitis)

What Causes Graves's Disease: My Own Clinical Research

Not *every* genetically predisposed individual (not even twins) develops an autoimmune disease. We cannot do anything about genetics anyway. Are there some other factors responsible for autoimmune dysfunction and can they be treated? As an endocrinologist, I was curious about these questions. What I discovered is amazing!

In all of my patients with autoimmune diseases, including Graves' Disease, I discovered the following three factors play a *crucial* role in causing an autoimmune disease. What is even more exciting is that all of these factors are treatable.

Treatable Factors That Cause Graves' Disease

1. Worrying.

2. High Carbohydrate diet.

3. Vitamin D deficiency.

1. Worrying

I found that each and every one of my patients with Graves' Disease (and other autoimmune diseases as well) *worries* a lot. How can worrying cause autoimmune dysfunction?

Normally, your immune system is designed to deal with threats, let's say an invading virus. When faced with an army of viruses, your immune system recognizes these invading biologic agents as foreign and recruits an army of its own white cells, called lymphocytes. Think of these activated lymphocytes as soldiers called to duty. A *battle* takes place between the army of the viruses and your activated lymphocytes. If you win, you get over the viral illness. Then, these activated lymphocytes are sent back to the barracks. No more threat, no more need for the army of the activated lymphocytes.

Well, when you *worry* excessively, you are basically *afraid* that something bad may happen. In other words, your mind perceives a threat, *albeit a* virtual threat. The immune system *reacts* to the threat: virtual or real - It doesn't matter. An army of the activated lymphocytes is recruited. Think of the activated lymphocytes as *hyped up* soldiers looking for the enemy, but there is *no* enemy. The threat is *virtual*, but they have to attack someone. So they start to attack your body's own cells, such as thyroid cells. Think of the thyroid cells as innocent bystanders, who get scared and start to run after seeing soldiers carrying guns. This simply *energizes* the soldiers. They *mistakenly* believe they have found the enemy and ask for reinforcement. They unleash their *weaponry* in the form of antibodies, such as Thyroid Stimulating Immunoglobulins or TSI, which are in fact, antibodies directed at TSH receptors in the thyroid cells. That's why these antibodies are also called TSH Receptor Antibodies or Thyrotropin Receptor Antibodies (TRAB.)

In other words, activated lymphocytes get control of the perceived enemy's targets, in this case the TSH receptors on the thyroid cells, through the production of TSH receptor antibodies. After seizing these receptors, these TSH receptor antibodies command the thyroid cells to produce an *increased* amount of thyroid hormone.

Normally, your pituitary gland *regulates* the production of thyroid hormone by the thyroid gland. For example, if your pituitary gland detects thyroid hormone to be low in the blood, it places an *order* to produce more thyroid hormone. Your pituitary gland sends this *message* for the increased production of thyroid hormone as an increased amount of TSH. On the other hand, if your pituitary gland detects thyroid hormone to be high, it cuts back on the *order* by reducing the amount of TSH. In this way, there is a fine regulation of the thyroid hormone production, the pituitary being the <u>high command</u>.

In the case of Graves' disease, once the antibodies from the activated lymphocytes seize *control* of the perceived enemy's factory of thyroid hormone production, they also *disrupt* the normal control from the high command, the pituitary gland. The pituitary keeps sending the message to the thyroid gland *not* to produce any more thyroid hormone, since there is *too* much thyroid hormone in the blood already. That's why you have very low or even undetectable TSH on your blood test. However, the *besieged* thyroid cells don't receive this important message. Why? Because now, they are under the command of the *new* boss: <u>TSH receptor antibodies</u>, which completely *disregard* the important message from the pituitary gland. That's why the thyroid cells continue to produce increased amounts of thyroid hormone, although your blood already contains a large amount of thyroid hormone. In other words, the normal, *logical* high command of the pituitary gets replaced by the new, *illogical* command by these antibodies, who *hijack* your thyroid gland and tell it what to do.

TSH receptors are also present in the fatty/connective tissues in the eyeball, as well as in the connective tissue in the skin (1). Activated lymphocytes in patients with Graves' disease *chase* TSH receptors as perceived enemies and end up mounting an attack on the fatty-connective tissue present in the orbit of the eye and in the skin of susceptible individuals. This is how you may develop Graves' orbitopathy and/or dermopathy. (More on this later in the book.)

2. High Carbohydrate Diet

Extensive scientific studies have clearly established that diet plays an important role in the causation and progression of autoimmune diseases. But how? Certain genetically predisposed individuals are *not* able to digest starches and sugars properly. The partially digested starches and sugars provide fertile grounds for bacteria and yeast to thrive in the intestines, causing "bacterial overgrowth." The byproducts of these micro-organisms cause inflammation of the intestinal walls, making them more permeable. Large molecules of partially digested food can then leak into the blood stream. This is called *Leaky Gut Syndrome*, which in turn, activates your immune system. The activated lymphocytes then start to attack various organs in the body, giving rise to a variety of clinical symptoms. In the case of Graves' Disease, these activated lymphocytes can produce special antibodies, called Thyroid Stimulating Antibodies, which attach themselves to the TSH receptor on the thyroid cells and force them to produce a large amount of thyroid hormone, which causes overactive thyroid or hyperthyroidism.

Therefore, starches and sugars play an important role in causing and perpetuating autoimmune diseases including Graves' Disease.

3. Vitamin D Deficiency

Vitamin D is actually not a vitamin, but a hormone. Vitamin D is produced in the skin from 7-dehydrocholesterol (pro-vitamin D3) which is derived from cholesterol. Here is evidence that cholesterol is not all bad, contrary to what most people think these days. The fact is that cholesterol is a precursor for most hormones in your body.

Type B Ultraviolet rays (UVB) from the sun act on pro-vitamin D3 and convert it into pre-vitamin D3, which is then converted into vitamin D3. Medically speaking, we call it cholecalciferol. Vitamin D3 then leaves the skin and gets into the blood stream where it is carried on a special protein called a vitamin D-binding protein.

Through blood circulation, vitamin D3 reaches various organs in the body. In the liver, vitamin D3 undergoes a slight change in its chemical structure. At that point, it is called 25, hydroxy cholecalciferol or 25 (OH) Vitamin D3 (or calcifediol). It is then carried through the blood stream to the kidneys where it goes through another change in its chemical structure. At that point, it is called 1,25 dihydroxy cholecalciferol or 1,25 $(OH)_2$ vitamin D3 (or calcitriol). This is the active form of vitamin D. It gets in the blood stream and goes to various parts of the body and exerts its actions. That is why vitamin D is really a hormone.

Vitamin D plays an important role in the *normal* functioning of the immune system. There is a strong scientific evidence to incriminate low vitamin D as an important factor in the causation of autoimmune diseases such as rheumatoid arthritis (2), lupus (3), fibromyalgia (4), multiple sclerosis (5,6), and Type 1 diabetes (7). In an experimental study from UCLA School of Medicine, vitamin D deficiency was found to cause Graves' Disease (8).

My clinical experience at the Jamila Diabetes and Endocrine Medical Center shows vitamin D to be low in every patient with autoimmune diseases, including patients with Graves' disease.

Footnote

As I was writing this book, I did some exploration on the internet and found this fascinating story:

Dr. Caleb Hillier Parry, a British physician, was a busy family physician who was a keen observer. In 1786, he first described a case of hyperthyroidism, what we now know as Graves' Disease. That's why there is an interest to change the name of Graves' Disease to its true pioneer and call it Parry's Disease.

In his original description, Dr. Parry describes the case of a woman, Elizabeth S., who was thrown out of her wheelchair while coming downhill fast. She was not seriously hurt, but terribly frightened. In 2 weeks time, she noticed swelling of her thyroid gland and symptoms of hyperthyroidism. A brilliant example of how acute, fearful stress can trigger Graves' Disease.

References:

1. Williams GR. Extrathyroidal expression of TSH receptor. *Ann Endocrinol* (Paris). 2011 Apr;72(2):68-73

2. Merlino LA, Curtis J, Mikuls TR et al. Vitamin D intake is inversely associated with rheumatoid arthritis: results from the Iowa Women's Health Study. *Arthritis Rheum* 2004;50:72-77.

3. Kamen DL, Cooper GS, Bouali H, et al. Vitamin D deficiency in systemic lupus erythematosus. *Autoimmune Rev* 2006;5:114-117

4. Huisman AM, White KP, Algra A, et al. Vitamin D levels in women with systemic lupus erythematosus and fibromyalgia. *J Rheumatol* 2001;28:2535-2539.

5. Hayes CE. Vitamin D. a natural inhibitor of multiple sclerosis. *Proc Nutr Soc.* 2000;59(4):531-535.

6. Raghuwanshi A, Joshi SS, Christakos S. Vitamin D and multiple sclerosis. *J Cell Biochem.*2008;105(2):338-343.

7. Hypponen E, Laara E, Reunanen A, et al. Intake of vitamin D and risk of Type 1 diabetes: a birth-cohort study. *Lancet* 2001;358:1500-1503.

8. Misharin A, Hewison M et al. Vitamin D deficiency modulates Graves' hyperthyroidism induced in BALB/c mice by thyrotropin receptor immunization. *Endocrinology.* 2009, 150(2):1051-1060.

9. Parry CH. Collection from the unpublished medical papers of the late Caleb Hillier Parry, M.D.,F.R.C. Vol.2,.p 111. London, Underwoods, 1825.

Chapter 9

My 5 Step, New Strategy To Treat Graves' Disease: A Scientific, Sensible And Effective Approach

Is it possible to treat Graves' disease effectively in a scientific manner by treating its root cause, the autoimmune process? I asked this question early in my career as an endocrinologist. Once I fully understood what causes the autoimmune disease process in a patient with Graves' Disease, I set up a strategy to treat the factors that cause the autoimmune process. Did it work?

I am quite excited to report this strategy has worked extremely well in my patients. The vast majority (more than 95%) of my patients have been able to *avoid* radioactive iodine or surgery and their *horrendous* consequences. That's why I decided to write this book, so I could share this vital information with my readers.

My new strategy to treat Graves' disease consists of Five steps:

- Freedom from worrying.
- Special Diet for Graves' Disease.
- Vitamin D supplementation.
- Vitamin B12 supplementation.
- Judicious use of anti-thyroid drugs.

In the next five chapters, I explain each step in detail.

Chapter **10**

Freedom from Worrying

What I discovered is that patients with Graves' Disease and other autoimmune diseases *worry* a lot about every little thing. Often, they are *afraid* of this or that.

When you worry, your body thinks that it is under attack. Therefore, your immune system gets into a high alert state to fight off the offending agent, but there is no one to fight off! Confused, it starts to attack its own organs, causing a variety of diseases. If it attacks the thyroid gland, you can develop Graves' Disease (which results in hyperthyroidism) or Hashimoto's Thyroiditis (which can result in hypothyroidism).

Why Do We Worry?

Use logic and you realize the underlying cause of "worrying" is fear.
Fear comes in many forms. Some examples:

1. Fear of the Future

You may be afraid something *bad* may happen in the *future*, based upon your *past* experience or the experience of others that you have heard about through chatting, the news media, internet, books or knowledge of history. You *do not* want it to happen to you ever, because it was (or could be) so painful. The mere thought that it may happen *triggers* a wave of fear and anxiety in you. This leads to "What If Syndrome" or "What May Syndrome" or "What Will I Do Syndrome."

Here are some examples:

- What if I have another attack of asthma, colitis or a migraine headache?
- What if Wall Street takes a nose-dive again?
- What if I get stung by a bee again?
- What if I miss my important meeting?
- What if I develop diabetes and die a miserable death like my mother?
- What happens if global warming continues?
- What happens if some bad people come into power?
- What if there is a severe shortage of my thyroid medication, insulin or water supply?
- What will I do if run out of my retirement money?
- What will I do if my mother/father/children are not around any more?
- What will I do if someone breaks into my house in the middle of the night?
- What will I do if I have no money, no insurance, no friends?
- What will I do if someone tries to rob me or rape me?
- What if my boyfriend/girlfriend cheats on me?

2. Fear of Losing

Often, you are afraid to lose what you have. For example:

- Fear of losing your job, business, money, stocks, retirement.
- Fear of losing your spouse, parents, children, siblings, friends, pets.
- Fear of losing your looks.
- Fear of losing your house, car, jewelry, photo-albums.
- Fear of losing your respect, credibility, position, reputation.
- Fear of losing your professional license.
- Fear of losing your power.
- Fear of losing your composure, self-control.
- Fear of losing your No. 1 spot.
- Fear of losing your health.

- Fear of losing your independent living.
- Fear of losing your life.
- Fear of losing your religion, culture, country.
- Fear of losing elections.
- Fear of losing planet earth.

3. Fear of Failure

You may be afraid you won't be able to live up to expectations.
For example:

- Fear of failing as a good mother/ father.
- Fear of failing as a good child.
- Fear of failing as a good brother/ sister.
- Fear of failing as a good friend.
- Fear of failing as a good teacher/ student.
- Fear of failing as a good boss /employee.
- Fear of failing as a good doctor, teacher, lawyer, etc.
- Fear of failing as a good guru, enlightened person, yoga instructor.
- Fear of failing as a good driver, pilot or captain of the boat.
- Fear of failing as a patriot, soldier or general.
- Fear of failing as a good citizen, journalist, moral person.
- Fear of failing as a good social, religious or political leader.
- Fear of failing as a nice person, who keeps his/her appointment, commitments, promises, wedding vows.

4. Fear of Social Situations

You may be fearful of humiliation and criticism. For example:

- Fear of rejection, social outcast.
- Fear of embarrassment.
- Fear of shame.
- Fear of insults.
- Fear of being late.

- Fear of premature ejaculation, sexual performance or impotence.

5. Fear of Punishment And Sufferings

Fear also arises when you are afraid of punishment and painful sufferings. For example:

- Fear of being caught: with a prostitute, cheating, bribing, stealing, swindling, having sex, being nude, watching pornography, masturbating, living as an illegal immigrant, driving without a license, practicing without a license.
- Fear of monetary penalty.
- Fear of social boycott.
- Fear of imprisonment.
- Fear of torture.
- Fear of deportation, poverty and its associated sufferings.
- Fear of sufferings from disease and disability.

6. Fear of Lack Of Control/Vulnerability

You may be afraid of being vulnerable. Here are some examples:

- Fear of the unknown.
- Fear of the outcome.
- Fear of unpreparedness.
- Fear of lack of knowledge.

Ultimate Freedom From Fear

In order to be free of fear, first you need to find out what is the root cause of fear, instead of running away from fear and finding a quick fix. The quick fix approach will be superficial, a band-aid that won't work effectively in the long run. That's why anti-anxiety medications may provide you with temporary relief of symptoms arising out of fear, but they do not get rid of fear at its roots. Many other techniques to conquer your fear may suppress your fear for a while, but deep down you continue to be fearful.

So, what's the root cause of fear?

The Root Cause Of Fear

Use common sense, and you will see that fear is an emotion, triggered by a "frightening thought." The emotion of fear then influences your thought process, which becomes more frightful. Then, it generates more emotions of fear. Thus, a vicious cycle sets in: thoughts generate fear and fear generates more thoughts.

This vicious cycle can induce some neurochemical changes in your brain, as well as release of the hormones adrenaline and cortisol from the adrenal glands. All of these chemical changes give rise to manifestations of fear, which range from insomnia, anxiety and phobias to panic attacks, allergies and autoimmune disorders.

What Is The Basis Of Thoughts?

It is pretty clear that thoughts give rise to fear. Where do thoughts come from? While pondering over this question one day, I made a simple, yet profound observation. We humans, always think in terms of a language. For example, if you know English and no other language, you will always think in English, not in Chinese, French or Hindi. Just observe it right now, yourself.

In order to think, you need to know a language. Therefore, language is the basis of thoughts.

What Is The Basis Of Language?

Obviously, the next question is where does the language come from? You are not born with it, right? You learn it as you grow up in a society. You learn it from your parents, teachers, siblings, friends and various tools such as books, electronic devices and sometimes, certain other techniques.

What Is A Language?

Let's use common sense and explore what is a language. It is a means to communicate with each other. A language is comprised of words, right? And each word has a concept attached to it. In reality, every word is a sound. For example, listen to a language you don't know. All you will hear is sounds, sounds that make no sense.

In order to make sense, you need to know the concepts attached to the sounds. In this way, we can say that a word consists of a <u>sound</u> and an attached <u>concept</u>. Even written language has <u>concepts</u> attached to words. Even Sign language has <u>concepts</u> attached to signs.

What Is The Basis Of Concepts?

Let's use common sense and find out where concepts come from. Concepts are the creation of a society, aren't they? When you grow up in a society, your parents teach you the language of that society. They utter a sound and point to a person or some object. They keep repeating it until you make a *connection* between that sound and the person or object. For example: As a baby, you hear the sound Mama as your mother points a finger towards herself. After a lot of repetition, you make a connection between the sound and the person. She is no longer another life form, but Mama. She provides you with food, comfort and warmth. You get *attached* to her. Later, she provides you with toys, gifts, friends, cupcakes, cookies, money and so on. You get more and more attached to "your Mama."

As you grow up in a society, you are *bombarded* with concepts that the society has created, such as the concepts of success, failure, achievement, money, fame, desirable, undesirable, morality, etiquette, responsibility, culture, customs, religion, nationality, past, future, security. Based on these concepts, certain thoughts may arise, such as thoughts of losing, being a failure, an outcast, punishment, suffering, the future, insecurity, etc. All of these thoughts create a huge amount of fear.

Sooner or later, you are introduced to the concept of death. Then a thought runs through your head - What if my Mama dies? This triggers a wave of fear and anxiety throughout your body.

As you grow up in a society, you also acquire a lot of information, all of which is based on language. In other words, you need a language to understand any information. Your society provides you with this information, usually in the form of the news media, books, internet, etc. In this way, you acquire a lot of information about some dreadful event that happened hundreds *if* not thousands of miles away. Perhaps, that tragic incident happened years or even centuries ago, before you were even born. Based on all of this fearful information in your head, some new thoughts arise. "What if it happens to me?" "What will I do?" All of these thoughts then trigger a lot of fear in you.

Who Is Thinking?

If you pay attention, you realize it is always "I" who is afraid of this or that. It is the "I" who is thinking. Therefore, it is the "I" who is at the root of all of the fear. Who is this "I"? We need to figure this out, if we truly want to be free of fear.

The "I"

Who is this "I" that is thinking and is fearful? You may reply, "Oh! It's me." Really?

Let's take a look at this "I". Can you show me where is it? It's in your head, isn't it? It's an abstraction, an illusion, a phantom. It is a *virtual* entity in your head that *steals* your identity. It is not the "true" you at all. Why do I say that? Because you are not born with this. In order to know your "True, Original Self," observe little babies, just a day or so old. I had the opportunity to be in charge of a well-baby nursery in my early career as a doctor and observed about sixty babies every day. Later, I had the wonderful experience of having my own baby.

When you observe little babies, you see that as soon as their basic physical needs are met (ie. a full stomach, a clean diaper and a warm blanket), they are *joyful* from within! They *smile* and go to sleep. They have no *past* or *future*. They are *not* worried if mom will be around for the next feed. If they did, they wouldn't be able to go to sleep. They don't think. Hence, there is no concept, no future and consequently, no *fear* and no *worries*. That's why they have no problem going to sleep. They are so *vulnerable*, but *fear* remains miles away. There is a total *lack of control,* but *no fear* whatsoever.

Once their stomach is full, they *don't* want any more food. If you were to force more food than they need, they would regurgitate. They eat to satisfy their hunger and that's all. *Wanting more* does not exist and that's why they are so *content*. You could feed them breast milk, cow's milk or formula. To them, it doesn't matter as long as it agrees with their stomach and satisfies their hunger.

They don't say "I don't like your milk, Mom. I like formula milk better." You won't hear, "Mom, you wrapped me in a pink blanket with butterflies on it. I'm a boy. Therefore, I need a blue blanket with pictures of dinosaurs on it."

They are joyful just looking around. They truly *live in the moment*. They do it spontaneously without making an effort to live in the Now.

Why do I say newborn babies don't think? Because, you always think in terms of a language. Newborns know *no* language. Hence, they don't think. They also have no concepts. Why? Because concepts arise out of language. No language - no concepts.

Newborn babies don't like or dislike someone because of their color, religion, nationality or wealth. That's because they have not acquired any *concepts* about religion, nationality, history or money. *Concepts* do not exist at all. *Likes and dislikes* do not exist. There are no *preferences or judgments*. No *embarrassment or shame.*

No fear, no anger, no hate, no wanting more, no prejudices...
Just pure joy, contentment and peace. Every moment is *fresh, pristine* and *new. This is the True Human Nature.* I like to call it the "True Self," the self that you and I and everyone else on the planet is born with.

Now let's see what happens to this fearless, joyful and peaceful baby.

The Acquired Self

Gradually, another self develops as you grow up in a society. This, we can call the *Acquired Self.* You acquire it as a result of *psychosocial conditioning*, from your parents, your school and then, your society in general.

As you grow, this Acquired Self gets bigger and bigger. It gets in the driver seat, pushing the True Self onto the passenger side and later, into the back seat and eventually, into the trunk.

As a grown up, all you see is this Acquired Self. You identify with this Acquired Self. *That's who you think you are.* This becomes the virtual "I" sitting in your head. Your identity gets *hijacked* by the Acquired Self. Instead of seeing the hijacker for what it is, you think that's who you are. How ironic!

This Acquired Self is the basis for all of your stress, including worries. It reacts to outside triggers, which it calls stressors and blames them for your stress. In fact, it is the Acquired Self who reacts to triggers and creates stress for you. In this way, the source of all stress actually resides insides you. It is good to know this very basic fact. Why? Because if the source of stress is inside you, so is the solution.

This Acquired Self torments you and creates stress even when there is no stressful situation. It conveniently creates *hypothetical* situations (the What If Syndrome) to make you fearful. I like to call it a *monster*, as it is quite frightening and appears strong, but in the end, it is really virtual.

Sadly, you don't even have a clue what's going on, because you completely identify with the Acquired Self, the mastermind behind all of your stress. You could call it the *enemy within*.

Unfortunately, you're completely out of touch with your True Self, the source of true joy, contentment and inner peace. In the total grip of the monstrous Acquired Self, you suffer and suffer and create stress not only for yourself, but for others as well.

The Composition Of Your Acquired Self

At the core of your Acquired Self is the virtual, conceptual "I" you *mistakenly* think you are. Around this "I," there are layers and layers of concepts, information and knowledge, downloaded into your growing Acquired Self. Some examples: My parents, My teachers, My friends, My school, My career, My goals, My car, My house, My beauty, My jewelry, My ancestors, My accomplishments, My culture, My town, My country, My religion, My past, My future.

The Making Of The Virtual "I"

Where does the virtual "I" come from? It is actually a <u>concept</u> that gets downloaded into your head. It starts from home. Your parents carefully select a <u>label</u> for you. They call it your name, which is basically a sound. Your parents utter this sound as they point towards you. After doing it repeatedly, they finally succeed in drilling into your head that you are indeed Peter, Lisa or Susan. At the same time, they also drill in the concepts of Mama and Dada.

As you grow up in a society, you acquire more and more concepts, which circle around the concept of "I," just like the layers of an onion.

How Your Acquired Self Creates Fear For You

Once your Acquired Self *steals* your identity, it *runs* your life. Then, you experience life through the *filters* created by your Acquired Self. These filters come from concepts, knowledge, information and experiences. The experiences can be your own as well as the experiences of others (virtual experiences for you), in the form of stories and opinions you saw in newspapers, books, magazines, TV or the internet or heard from friends and family.

Basically, your Acquired Self wants to live a very secure life. It wants security. Why? Because it is *inherently* insecure. It is *not* real. It is virtual, a phantom, an illusion, but it thinks it is real and it wants to live forever. Pretty crazy, isn't it?

In order to be safe, your Acquired Self *interprets* every experience (real experience or virtual experience. It doesn't matter) based on the information stored in it and judges the experience to be good or bad, which triggers an emotion, good or bad. Then, it *stores* the entire experience along with the triggered emotion into your *memory* box, where it stays *alive*, even years later. This is how your mind creates your *memories* or the <u>past</u>.

Experiences which are labeled good, your Acquired Self wants *more* of and the ones labeled bad, it wants to *run* away from. This is the basis of psychological *attachment* and *avoidance*.

Your Acquired Self gets very *attached* to good experiences, such as praise and validation, which provides a *temporary* relief from its insecurity. That's why your Acquired Self gets attached to the concepts of *money*, *power* and *success*, all of which bring it praise and validation. With money and power, it can acquire *possessions,* which enhances its *ego* and provides *temporary* validation and relief from insecurity.

Your Acquired Self is often very attached to the concept of beauty. Why? Because it provides praise, validation and temporary relief from insecurity. However, you end up spending a lot of time and money to look beautiful. You become a frequent visitor to beauty parlors, shopping malls and may even see a plastic surgeon to enhance/preserve your looks. You get stuck with huge bills, which create more stress. Then, one day you may notice wrinkles on your face or excessive hair loss, which may push a *panic* button. In my practice, I have had patients wanting to be seen on an urgent basis because they noticed clumps of hair falling out of their head during their morning shower. They act like it's the end of the world.

Your Acquired Self also gets *praise* from family, friends and fans regarding its success, fame and accomplishments. It wants more and more of these experiences. It also feels *validated* when it is related, bonded or responsible for someone. For example, if you own a pet, it *validates* the existence of you as an owner and provides your Acquired Self a temporary relief from insecurity. That's why it doesn't want to ever *lose* its pets, family, friends and fans. *Even the idea of losing them rips through the paper thin layer of security and stirs up deep-seated, inherent insecurity which triggers a huge amount of fear.*

Your Acquired Self also seeks validation through conceptual identities such as a doctor, lawyer, teacher, political, social or religious leader, movie star, employee of a certain company, citizen of a certain country, member of a certain social, political or religious group, etc. That's why even the thought of losing its virtual identity creates a huge amount of fear. This is why you are so afraid of the possibility of losing your professional license, career, citizenship, elections, etc.

Your Acquired Self does not *ever* want to *lose* anything or anyone that is "Mine." That would mean losing a part of "Mine." How terrible that would be? That's why it is afraid of losing possessions. The more possessions you have as "My, Mine," the more you *fear* losing them and the more you try to protect them. You may end up living in a gated community to protect your belongings. Even news of someone getting robbed creates a lot of fear for you.

In addition, your Acquired Self wants to *avoid* unpleasant experiences, such as failure, punishment, loneliness, humiliation, poverty, aging, disease and death at all costs. *Even the thought of such unpleasant experiences triggers intense fear.*

In order to be secure, your Acquired Self also uses the following strategy. It has been conditioned to *learn* from its past. So it uses its past experiences or even the experiences of others that it has heard about and creates *hypothetical,* frightening situations, which is the basis of "What If, What May Syndrome." Then, it tries to find solutions, which is the basis of "What Will I Do Syndrome."

In reality, those situations don't exist at all. In other words, your Acquired Self is so *insecure* and *afraid* of its own death, that it creates all *possible,* dreadful case scenarios and tries to *figure out* how it can *escape* its death in every possible way. In doing so, it creates tons of *unnecessary* fear for you.

Your Acquired Self also quickly wants to interpret every situation it encounters and every person it meets, based upon the stored information. Why? Because it wants to feel secure. Often, it will judge a person to be safe or unsafe, based upon their appearance, without even exchanging a word. Often, it doesn't want to take any chances, so it won't interact with anyone it doesn't know.

You may remember "don't talk to strangers," from your childhood. You also want to make sure to download this very important message into the growing Acquired Self of your children. Maybe you read a story about some girl who got abducted by a stranger in a place you know nothing about. It rips through your feeling of security. Ironically, it reinforces your self-fulfilling prophecy of being "fearful of strangers." Obviously, you don't hear or pay attention to the countless safe encounters with strangers.

Your Acquired Self also wants to know everything about the future in order to feel safe. Otherwise, it suffers from the fear of the unknown.

Your Acquired Self is very afraid of your death, because it fears its own death with your death. Therefore, any thought about death triggers a huge amount of fear.

Be The Master Of Your Acquired Self, Not Its Slave

The root cause of your fear and all other stress actually resides inside you - your Acquired Self. Therefore, the solution must also reside inside you.

In summary, your Acquired Self is the virtual, conceptual "I" you *mistakenly* think you are. It's consists of "My name, My personality, My beliefs, My past, My future, My parents, My children, My teachers, My friends, My students, My school, My career, My goals, My accomplishments, My failures, My culture, My town, My country, My religion, etc. It is a virtual *entity* sitting inside you, but it is not the *true* you. It *steals* your identity. It controls your *thoughts*, *emotions* and *actions*. The Acquired Self is the basis of the "Busy Mind," a *constant* stream of thoughts. Then, thoughts *provoke* emotions and emotions *taint* your thoughts. A vicious cycle of thought-emotion-thought sets in. This is the basis of worrying, anxiety, anger, frustrations, hate, love, revenge, jealousy, guilt, sadness, depression, selfishness, greed, ego, self-righteousness, expectations, judging, hypocrisy, embarrassment and shame. Then, *actions* arise out of these thoughts and emotions, which often cause stress for you and others. The actions may be verbal, written or physical.

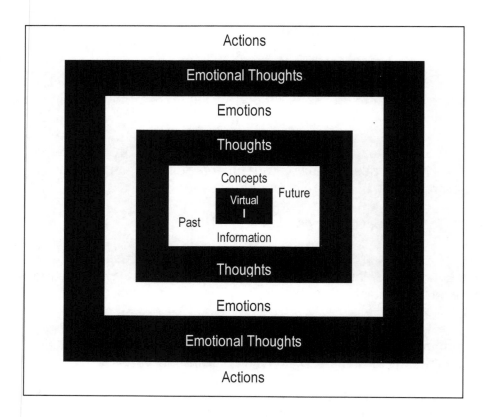

The Acquired Self

How To Rise Above Your Acquired Self

First of all, you have to see your Acquired Self as separate from you. Only then, can you see it for what it is. However, if you continue to *identify* with your Acquired Self, you can *never* see its true colors. As long as you and your Acquired Self are *stuck* together, obviously you can *never* be free of it.

In order to *free* yourself from your Acquired Self, you have to see it in action. When you're in the grip of your Acquired Self, you *immediately* react to *triggers*. We can call it <u>auto-pilot</u> mode. These automatic reactions often cause more stress for you and others. Later on, when you come to your senses, you often *regret* what you said or did.

1. Don't React Immediately!

The *first step* to *separate* yourself from your Acquired Self is to *not* let it automatically control your actions. Stop for a moment and *pause* before you *react* to what you read, hear or watch.

2. Shift Your Awareness/Attention To The Now

Shift your attention to the *Now*. What is Now? Now is *not* what is in your head, but what is in front of your eyes. It is your <u>field of awareness</u>.

Pause for a moment right now and pay attention to what you see, what you hear, what you smell, what you taste and what you touch. Don't think, just observe. Experience what's in your field of awareness.

In general, when we see, we only pay attention to objects without paying any attention to the *space* in which everything is. Without space, there would be no objects. So when you see objects, also be aware of the space which gives rise to all objects.

In the same way, when you listen, also pay attention to the *silence*, without which there would be no sound.

Use your eyes and ears and be aware of space, *silence* and *stillness*, which gives rise to all objects, events and sounds.

In addition to your outer field of awareness, you also have an *inner field of awareness.* This inner field of awareness is your *Original Self*.

It is vibrant, full of immense energy, joy and inner peace. No words can accurately describe it... But it can be felt. It is Real and not a concept. That's why your Acquired Self, which consists of concepts, cannot understand it. You can feel your inner field of awareness simply by calming your busy mind and taking your attention inside you.

In fact, your outer field of awareness is an extension of your inner field of awareness. It is <u>one</u> field of awareness... And that is what the Now is! I made this arbitrary distinction of inner and outer field of awareness just to communicate with you. That's all!

Practice to be aware of the Now around you and inside you. Then, you can easily *shift* your attention to the *Now* as soon as you realize your thoughts and emotions have taken over you.

The moment you switch your attention to the Now, you are free of your thoughts and their associated emotions. In other words, you are free of your Acquired Self. *Instantaneously,* you will feel *relief* from fear or any other stressful emotion. That's how powerful this seemingly simple step is. A moment later, your attention may again be *sucked* up by thoughts and emotion. Simply keep shifting your attention/awareness into the Now.

Your Acquired Self needs your *attention* to thrive. That's why it *sucks* up your attention/awareness most of the time. However, you have the power to *switch* gears and *divert* your attention/awareness to the Now. Without your attention/awareness, your Acquired Self can no longer survive. As long as your attention/awareness is in the Now, you are free of the Acquired Self.

Remember this phrase: <u>Keep your mind where your body is</u>.

While fully aware of the Now, feel and watch the drama your Acquired Self creates. Don't run away from it. After a little while, it will settle down.

<u>Example:</u>

You're stuck in traffic on your way to the airport. You start worrying. "What if I miss my flight and then I'll miss my interview for this job I really want and my best chance to get this dream job will evaporate" and on and on. You get so *fearful* from the drama that your Acquired Self creates, that you may end up having chest pain and find yourself heading to a hospital... <u>Or</u> you can choose to shift your attention from thoughts to the Now: Watch the car in front of you, the cars to each side, the median of the freeway, the electric poles seemingly running backwards, the sky, the clouds, etc. Also pay attention to your breathing, which is a continuous act in the Now. Chances are pretty good that you will arrive at the airport safely, certainly without any fear or high blood pressure. You may or may not be late. If you are late, you will deal with it. Therefore, live in the Now, stay in reality and you won't have any fear.

Caution:

Be careful *not* to confuse *attention* with *concentration*. Attention is simple awareness, that's all! It is there automatically, without any effort. On the other hand, concentration and discipline require a lot of effort and are quite stressful by themselves.

3. Use Logic - Common Sense

Now take the next step: use *logic*, the most wonderful tool we humans have. Why? Because the Acquired Self is always *illogical* and can't stand the blazing *torch* of logic. Therefore, use logic and see the *true colors* of your Acquired Self. See for yourself who is really at the root of fear and all other stress. See how *illogical* your Acquired Self is.

For example, your Acquired Self remains *worried* about the so called future. Use common sense and you'll see whatever your thoughts imply, may or may not happen... But certainly, it's not happening in the Now, in front of your eyes, right? Therefore, it's a phantom, an illusion. How can you really take care of a problem that doesn't even exist? If and when it happens, at "that time, the present moment," you'll be able to take *real* action, instead of the *virtual* action your Acquired Self keeps thinking about, which serves no purpose, but simply generates fear.

Another example: You are in your sixties and doing fine. Then one day, you read in the newspaper that someone important died of cancer. Your Acquired Self triggers a thought... What if I have cancer? This creates another thought of possibly losing your health, autonomy and ultimately dying. This creates a huge amount of fear. You start to feel your heart pounding. You feel uneasiness and anxiety. Then, you start wondering who'll take care of your wife if you die, which further worsens your fear and suddenly, you've got a full fledged panic attack.

Even in the midst of this panic attack, pause, take some deep breaths and start counting your breaths. Look around and see what is actually happening in front of you. Feel the space inside your chest. At the same time, feel the fear, but don't get consumed by it. Fully realize that it is your Acquired Self who is fearful. Your True Self, space, is untouchable. Then, use logic. Ask yourself: Do I have cancer at this moment? Am I losing my autonomy at this moment? You realize you really don't have any problems at this moment. Then, you also clearly see that it is actually your Acquired Self playing tricks with you by creating an imaginary future. The moment you clearly see the Acquired Self for what it is, an entity separate from you, it starts to lose its power over you. Using logic, you also tell your mind: "I will deal with any medical condition, if and when it arises." Make a mental note to discuss it with your doctor on your next visit or even write it down on a piece of paper. You will see fear completely evaporate and you can move on with your everyday life.

In addition, *acknowledge* the basic law of nature: if you are born, then one day you die. There are *no* exceptions to this rule. The Acquired Self however, does not want to die and wishes to live forever. Therefore, it makes death something you must avoid, cheat, conquer, etc. In this way, it creates a lot of *negativity* about death. In the grip of their Acquired Self, many people *worry* about death all their life and then one day they die. How sad!

Stop worrying and start living. You can do it once you are free of your Acquired Self.

Instead of worrying, take action in the present moment. For example, eat right, exercise regularly and take vitamin D every day. There's a good chance you won't develop asthma, colitis, cancer, diabetes, high blood pressure or heart disease. Even if you do develop any medical condition, you will be able to deal with it at that time.

However, if you just keep worrying and don't take any actions, chances are you may develop these diseases. Take real action in the present moment, instead of worrying about the results.

<u>Caution:</u>

Please be aware that I am using the word logic as the simple common sense that every human is born with. I am not using it as intellectualization, rationalization or reasoning.

4. Be Aware Of The Conceptual World We Live In

Have you ever pondered about the world we live in? If you take a fresh, logical look at the human world without preconceived notions, you will find that we live in a *conceptual world*, a *virtual world*, not a real world.

Because everyone around us lives in this collective conceptual, virtual world, we think it is real. Actually, we simply accept it as real and don't even bother investigating whether it is real or not.

For example, let's say you watch the Oscar Awards on TV. Through the goggles of the conditioned mind, (your Acquired Self), you see five actresses nominated for best actress. After a few moments of agony, everyone is told who wins *best actress of the year*. The winner is obviously thrilled and excited, but the other four feel defeated, though they try to force a fake smile. For the winner, the moment has finally arrived, the moment for which she has waited for years. She gets overwhelmed with emotions, but manages to deliver an tearful speech. Then, her moment is over. In few minutes, it is someone else going through similar emotions.

If you are a serious moviegoer, you have your own opinion as to *"who deserves to be the best actress."* If your choice wins, you are also *thrilled*, but if your choice loses, you will be *disappointed,* sometimes even *angry* and *bitter* about the *unfairness.*

You and the world calls it *entertainment*. You want more of it and the world is well equipped to provide you with more! Over the next several days, you enjoy seeing more and more about the whole event on the internet, TV, newspapers and magazines. You see stories about before and after parties, designer dresses, behind the scenes, etc., etc.

For the next few days, you even talk to your friends about the whole experience and have more fun. Actually, the more you know, the more you can impress your friends and the more special you feel about yourself.

Now, let's look at the whole event from an <u>unconditioned mind - someone without the Acquired Self</u>. Now, what you see is a person coming on stage to receive a shiny peace of metal. Holding that piece of metal in her hands, she gets very emotional, her eyes become tearful and her voice chokes. She says a few words and then everyone starts clapping. Why, you wonder?

Obviously, that piece of metal has a huge *concept* attached to it. The woman appearing on stage is not just a woman, but has a huge *concept* attached to her. The whole drama has a huge *concept* attached to it. *The entire concept reverberates with the concept in your head and in everyone else's head, about Oscars, actresses and actors, movies and the concepts of success, achievement, fame, wealth and glamour.*

In other words, your Acquired Self, the *Baby* Monster, gets fed by the *Papa* Monster of the society! That's why you enjoy it so much. For you and everyone else, it becomes real. Actually, you don't even question whether it is real or not. You watch and talk about it as if it was real.

It is interesting to know that you may be able to see the superficial, virtual nature of the part of the conceptual world that you are not attached to. For example, if you are attached to sports and not to movies, you may *not* be interested in watching the Oscars and may even realize their superficial nature, but you will not miss the Super Bowl, Wimbledon, the World Cup, the Olympics, etc. Each one of these words has huge concepts attached to them - the concepts of *victory, achievement, fame, wealth and glamour.*

If you use logic, you will find that most sports are about a ball that is kicked, thrown, carried and/or hit. The world does not see it that way. It sees these sports as a matter of *fight, victory, achievement, fame, glamour.*

By now, you may understand the virtual, conceptual nature of these events. However, you may say these are occasional events in your life. Well, take a close look at the usual activities of your daily life and you realize that most human activities are in the domain of the conceptual, virtual world.

Here are some examples: (*Let me make it very clear that I am making these observations using simple logic. I am not criticizing, putting down or making fun of any of these concepts. Of course, you don't have to agree with me.*)

The Internet, TV, newspapers and magazines obviously take you into the virtual, conceptual world. Many people start their day reading a newspaper or watching a morning show on TV. They glance through magazines or surf the internet during the day. In the evening, they usually watch TV or surf the internet. Most are hooked on TV or the internet for hours every day.

It's interesting to see some older people complain about young people wasting too much time on the internet, playing video games or texting. Meanwhile, they waste their time reading newspapers, watching TV and talking about politics or religion.

Everything you read in newspapers, magazines and books or watch on TV and the internet is conceptual and virtual, isn't it?

Everything in movies, stage shows, museums and art galleries is conceptual, isn't it? All pictures, paintings and statues are obviously conceptual.

All knowledge, whether history, mathematics, science, arts, geography or business is virtual and conceptual, isn't it? In this way, all of the educational system is conceptual.

Language itself is conceptual. Observe how every word carries a concept with it as we observed earlier in the book.

How about political and social systems? All are conceptual.

How about religious establishments? Those are all conceptual as well.

How about cultures, traditions and values? Those are all conceptual.

In reality, you see mountains, land, buildings, roads, trees, animals, sky, clouds and water. However, on a map you see continents, countries, states, provinces and cities - all conceptual.

How about marriage, romance, engagement, divorce? All are concepts, aren't they?

How about time? Seconds, minutes, hours, days, weeks, months and years. All conceptual. Different cultures have created different calendars.

How about national, religious and cultural holidays? All conceptual.

There are concepts attached to gold, platinum, jewels and diamonds. In fact, these are simply metals and rocks, but there are huge concepts attached to them.

How about money? This concept is so overwhelming that no one ever thinks of it as conceptual.

The Concept Of Money

Almost everyone is in the grip of the concept of money and the economy. For most people, it also creates a lot of worries.

What is the economy? It's a concept isn't it? You can not see the economy. You see currency, which itself is a concept. One Dollar, ten Euros, five Yen, a hundred pesos, fifty Rupees, etc.

If you give a 100 dollar bill to a one year old kid, she will probably put it in her mouth, chew on it or rip it apart. Why? Because she still has no concept of money. But give the same 100 dollar bill to her when she is a teenager and she will be thrilled to have it. Why? Because by now she has acquired the concept of money. In reality, it is a piece of paper, but of course, there is a concept attached to it.

Everyone wants to make money. Money itself is a concept, but people don't think of it that way. To them money is real. *"You can't do anything without money,"* you may argue, but that still does not make it real. *It may be necessary to some extent, but it is not real. To live in the conceptual world, you need money, but it still does not make it real.*

If you look deeper, you'll find that money is a way for humans to trade with each other. Not too long ago, people also used chickens, eggs, rice, etc. to purchase services from others. Animals don't do it.

Obviously, humans developed the *concept of trading.* The concept of trading came into being when humans started living in communities. For example, "I can exchange my eggs for your wheat." Initially, it served a purpose, but then it took over the human race. The concept of precious metals and money came into being. The more money (or precious metals) they had, the more they could buy. Initially, they bought things of necessity: food items, clothes, houses... But this was not enough. They wanted to acquire more and more. Why? Because society also created other concepts: The concepts of prestige, fame, glamour, enjoyment, entertainment, vacations and power. The more money you have, the more powerful, the more famous and the more prestigious you are. You can also have a high profile life-style.

With money, you can purchase various conceptual objects: the car of your dreams, your dream home, your dream vacation, etc. Money is no longer a means to buy the things of basic necessities, it is often used to *enhance* your ego, which is part of the Acquired Self.

"Wanting more" is the driving force behind the concept of money. There is never enough of it when you are in the grip of "wanting more." Even a billionaire tries to get more!

What's Wrong With Concepts?

There is nothing inherently wrong with concepts. It is only when they are not treated as concepts, but as reality, that they become problematic and create stress for you and others.

Use logic and you'll realize that *concepts are not reality and reality is not conceptual*... But most of humanity are lost in concepts and believe in them as if they were absolute truth. They get attached to them. They either love them (positive attachment) or hate them (negative attachment). Then, actions arise out of these attachments. Actions arising out of concepts create a huge amount of stress for you as well as everyone else.

Concepts also divide humans into groups. Each group believes their own concepts to be true. This obviously creates *conflict*. One group sees the other group as a *threat* to their collective belief system, which creates collective fear. This often leads to violence, verbal as well as physical and can even lead to battles and wars.

5. Utilize Your Acquired Self To Function In The World

The collective *conceptual* world, which we call the world, downloads a *conceptual* world into everyone's head, which is their Acquired Self. The two worlds are *extensions* of each other and *feed* each other. Basically, it is one big *conceptual* world.

Do Not start to hate your Acquired Self. In fact, your Acquired Self has its relative significance. It is your <u>tool</u> to function in the conceptual world, but obviously it is *not* you. The problem arises when you mistakenly believe your Acquired Self *is* you and you lose your true identity. Then, you are <u>enslaved</u> by your Acquired Self, which creates tons of stress for you and others. On the other hand, you need to *rise* above it and be its <u>master</u>, not its <u>slave</u>.

While interacting in the conceptual world, switch gears and shift some attention to your Acquired Self, but don't get overtaken by it. As soon as you don't need the assistance of your Acquired Self, switch gears and shift your attention to the Now.

In short, you are the *boss* of your attention. You can switch gears to shift your attention between your Acquired Self and the Now, back and forth. In this way, you can *function* in the conceptual world, without being enslaved by your Acquired Self.

6. Stress Free Living

With few exceptions, everyone is consumed by the *conceptual* world in their head, their Acquired Self and the collective, *conceptual* world, which we call the world.

As we observed, the conceptual world is full of stress. That's why people are so stressed out. They don't see any way out. They often *rationalize* their stressful living with statements such as "Oh, stress is part of life. There's nothing you can do about it." Then, they seek refuge in *escapes,* such as drugs, alcohol, partying, vacationing, gambling, etc, which provide only temporary relief and actually add more stress in the long run.

Once you *clearly* realize the *conceptual* nature of the "I" and the *conceptual* nature of the world, you are free of them. With this mental shift, a profound wisdom sinks in and your life becomes *stress free* automatically.

For example, you realize money is a concept. It helps you earn a living in the conceptual world, that's all! You earn money to meet the basic *necessities* of life such as food, shelter, clothing, transportation, etc. However, you clearly see the difference between "necessities" and "wanting." You realize it is the Acquired Self that has a never-ending list of "wanting," which is the basis of greed and lack of contentment.

You also clearly see how the Acquired Self boosts up its ego by pursuing certain respectable professions, by seeking fame, by living in a mansion, by acquiring certain possessions or by living a certain lifestyle. You also see the rat-race everyone is in to make more and more money and how it creates a huge amount of stress in their life.

Once you are free of wanting, greed and ego, you are content with whatever job or business you are in, as long as it provides you with the income to make a basic living. When you are not attached to your house, possessions or lifestyle, you are not worried about losing them.

In the grip of the conceptual world, a lot of people end up doing shady stuff to make more money. Then, they are *afraid* of being caught. Once you are free of greed, you obviously don't get into illegal practices to make more money. Then, you're *not* afraid of being caught, because you're not doing any shady stuff.

In addition, don't seek your *identity* through your profession, certain title or position. Then, you *don't* have thoughts about losing them and worries remains miles away.

As a student or parent of a student, you are no longer in a race to go to a prestigious college. As a student, you figure out what you're good at and pursue that particular field. It may or may not bring you a lot of money, but you are fine with this, because you are free of your Acquired Self and therefore, free of wanting, greed and ego. In this way, you don't have to go through tremendous worries such as "What if I don't get accepted at Harvard?"

You realize <u>rules are concepts</u>, but you also acknowledge their functional value. Therefore, you *follow* traffic rules, you *follow* campus rules, you *pay* your income tax and you *follow* the rules of your profession or business. In this way, you become a perfect law-abiding citizen. You have *nothing* to hide. Then, you have *no* fear of being caught.

You realize <u>marriage is a concept</u>, but you also realize its functional value and *follow* it as a part of living in a society. Free of your Acquired Self, you don't get into the mess of extra-marital affairs, which is the activity of the Acquired Self to enhance its ego or to escape from emotional pains. Obviously, if you don't have any affairs, you don't worry about being caught.

You realize <u>beauty is a concept</u>. Consequently, you *don't* worry if you lose a few hairs, if your hair start turning grey or if a wrinkle or a pimple appears on your face. You don't dye your hair, apply wrinkle cream or see a plastic surgeon. All the *worries* about side-effects of these dyes and creams, the high cost of plastic surgery and its possible side-effects automatically do not arise.

You recognize the conceptual nature of all sports, television shows and stocks Then, you *don't* worry about the loss of your team, the fate of your favorite TV show or the performance of your stocks.

You also realize all political, social and religious groups are virtual. Then, you *don't* take sides and *don't* worry if a certain group or party wins or loses.

You realize that internet, TV, newspapers and magazines keep you *trapped* in the conceptual world. Automatically, you don't spend much time on these activities. Then, you don't hear sensational, horrifying and dreadful news and stay free of unnecessary fear.

Once you realize the universal law of birth and death, you don't worry about death. In order to deal with a disease, you take the appropriate medicine and make necessary changes in your diet and exercise level. You realize you are alive until the moment you die. You realize life is to live and *not* to worry.

In short, *minimize* the conceptual world to bare <u>necessities</u>. In this way, you *free* up a lot of time to spend in the Real world, the Now, where there are no worries or any other type of stress... And it is *not* a boring life. Quite the opposite! Once you are in touch with your True Self, you tap into an *immense* source of <u>joy</u> and <u>inner peace</u>. Then, you have no need to seek thrill, excitement and entertainment.

That's how you live a life that is *joyful, peaceful* and completely *free* of fear as well as any other type of stress.

Chapter **11**

Diet for Graves' Disease

I recommend the following diet to my patients with Graves' disease.

WHAT NOT TO EAT

1. No Iodized Salt, Seafood, Seaweeds - No processed food.

Iodine is the essential ingredient of the thyroid hormone. In Graves' disease, the thyroid gland is already in high gear to produce thyroid hormone. For this reason, consumption of foods that are high in iodine can work as adding fuel to the fire. Therefore, avoid iodine-rich foods such as sea-food, seaweeds, and iodized salt. For taste, you can use sea-salt, which has low iodine content.

No canned foods, snack bars, or pre-cooked dinners. Have fresh foods, real foods and organic foods. The true nutritional value of a food (compared to what is written on the food label) is *lost* when it is processed, stored or frozen. In addition, many of these foods contain iodized salt.

Try to grow your own vegetables and fruits. In addition, use a local farmer's market to buy fruits and vegetables.

2. Eliminate Starches.

Starches are refined carbohydrates. What is a carbohydrate? In chemical terms, a carbohydrate consists of carbon, hydrogen and oxygen atoms.

As a dietary source, carbohydrates are divided into three types:

A. **Monosaccharides**, which consists of only <u>one</u> type of simple sugar, such as glucose or fructose. A monosaccharide does not require any further breakdown in the intestines before its absorption into the blood.

B. **Disaccharides,** which consists of <u>two</u> molecules of monosaccharide bonded together. For example, table sugar (sucrose) consists of glucose and fructose. Milk sugar (lactose) consists of glucose and galactose. A disaccharide requires further breakdown in the intestines before it can be absorbed into the blood. For example, sucrase, an enzyme in the intestinal wall, breaks down sucrose into glucose and fructose. Lactase, another enzyme in the intestinal wall, breaks down lactose into glucose and galactose.

C. **Polysaccharides,** which consists of hundreds to thousands of glucose molecules bonded together. During normal digestion, these polysaccharides are broken down into glucose, which is then absorbed into circulation. Digestion of polysaccharides is a complex process, which requires several digestive enzymes, including *maltase* in the small intestines.

A lot of individuals with Graves' disease cannot properly digest polysaccharides due to deficiency of the specific enzymes in the intestines. Partially digested polysaccharides become a great food for bacteria and yeast to grow, which leads to bacterial overgrowth and Leaky Gut Syndrome.

The main polysaccharides in our diets are <u>starches</u>. Therefore, **eliminate all starches from your diet.** <u>Starches include wheat, rice, oats, barley, rye, corn, potatoes, sweet potatoes and yams.</u>

There is another polysaccharide in our diet, called <u>cellulose</u>, which cannot be broken down in human intestines. Therefore, it does not become food for bacteria. Cellulose is our dietary fiber, an important ingredient for our health. It prevents rapid absorption of glucose, lowers cholesterol and forms bulk for the stools to prevent constipation.

It is interesting to note that in nature, plants contain carbohydrates as starch, cellulose and simple sugar, mainly fructose. After a plant is harvested, it goes through *processing* which gets rid of cellulose and what is left behind is starch. Therefore, we refer to starches as *refined* carbohydrates.

Some individuals with Graves' disease even develop loss of the intestinal villi, which are finger-like projections on the intestinal surface that are extremely important for digestion and absorption of polysaccharides. This is what we call Celiac disease or Gluten Sensitivity. There is a blood test to diagnose Celiac disease. The blood test aims to detect several special antibodies, called anti-tissue transglutaminase antibodies (tTGA) or anti-endomysium antibodies (EMA). Consider having this test done. If the test for Celiac disease is positive, then you should stay on a Gluten-free diet for the rest of your life. A Gluten-free diet means to eliminate all *wheat*, *barley*, *oats* and *rye* from your diet. You need to read labels carefully.

3. Say No to Sugar, Sugar Substitutes and Sugar Alcohols, but Yes to Honey

Say goodbye to sugar, even brown sugar and sugar-containing food items. Why? Sugar causes Leaky Gut Syndrome. This is how: A sugar molecule consists of glucose and fructose. During digestion, each sugar molecule has to be broken down into glucose and fructose by an enzyme called *sucrase*, before it can be absorbed from the intestines into the blood. A lot of individuals with Graves' disease do not have enough *sucrase* to digest sugar. Undigested sugar then serves as fertile ground for bacterial overgrowth in the intestine, which can lead to Leaky Gut Syndrome. As a result, there is unnecessary stimulation of the immune system, as I explained earlier.

You can use honey as a sweetener, because each honey molecule consists of only glucose. It does not require any breaking down in the intestines before its absorption into the blood.

Avoid artificial sweeteners such as Sucralose (Splenda), Saccharin (SugarTwin, Sweet'N Low), Aspartame (Equal, NutraSweet), Acesulfame (Sunett, Sweet One) and Neotame.

Also beware of <u>sugar alcohols</u> such as Sorbitol, Mannitol, Xylitol, Lactitol, Maltitol, Erythritol, Isomalt, Hydrogenated starch hydrolysates (HSH).

These artificial sweeteners are widely used in processed foods, including <u>sodas</u>, <u>powdered drink mixes</u>, <u>chocolate</u>, <u>cookies</u>, <u>cakes</u>, <u>chewing gum</u> and <u>candies</u>. These products are typically marketed as <u>sugar-free</u> and <u>low calorie</u>, which obviously has great appeal to the general public.

As a general rule of thumb, stay away from all processed food items. These are NOT natural, regardless what they claim. These are synthetic substances that may have started out from a natural substance, but the final product is far from anything that exists in nature. For example sucralose (in Splenda) is made when sugar is treated with trityl chloride, acetic anhydride, hydrogen chlorine, thionyl chloride and methanol in the presence of dimethylformamide, 4-methylmorpholine, toluene, methyl isobutyl ketone, acetic acid, benzyltriethlyammonium chloride, and sodium methoxide, according to the book *Sweet Deception*. This processing obviously makes sucralose unlike anything found in nature.

Artificial sweeteners and sugar alcohols can give rise to a number of side-effects, including gas and abdominal cramping. Why? Because these chemicals are usually not absorbed properly and become a fuel for bacterial overgrowth in the intestines. Some even cause neurologic symptoms such as confusion, headaches or dizziness. In addition, there are serious concerns about their long term safety.

Avoid any food item that contains <u>high fructose corn syrup</u>, as it provides fuel for the growth of bacteria in the intestines and contributes to Leaky Gut Syndrome. In addition, it also leads to obesity, diabetes, heart disease and liver damage.

<u>Here are some common food items you should avoid because they are loaded with starches and sugar or sugar substitutes.</u>

Bread, rice and pasta. Bread includes white bread, whole wheat bread, sourdough bread, French or Italian bread, bagels, croissants, biscuits, hamburger buns, rolls, pita, Indian naans, tortillas, tacos and many more similar bakery products.

Potato chips, Nachos, French fries.

Rice including white, brown as well as wild rice.

Waffles, pies, donuts, pancakes, pastries, cookies, candy and cakes.

Chocolate, cereals, pizza, chewing gum.

4. No Sodas, No Fruit Juices and No Alcohol.

Do not drink any sodas, even diet versions. Why? Because sodas are loaded with high fructose corn syrup and sugar. Diet sodas use artificial sweeteners and sugar alcohols.

Also avoid fruit juices, because fruit juices from grocery stores contains only a small amount of real juice and a lot of sugar water. Avoid even freshly squeezed, natural juice. Why? Because you end up consuming a <u>high</u> amount of natural sugar, fructose. For example, instead of eating just one whole orange, you will have to use 3-4 oranges to get about a cup of pure orange juice.

Instead of fresh juice, eat two to three Fresh fruit servings per day. Why? Because whole fruits not only contain sugar (fructose), but also the *pulp*, which slows down the absorption of sugar. That's why there is *less* of a rise in blood sugar level after eating a *whole fruit,* as compared to *fruit juice,* which causes a rapid rise in blood sugar level.

Avoid <u>alcoholic</u> beverages. Why? Because alcohol is a medically well known <u>toxin</u> for the liver, pancreas, brain and nerves. In addition, alcoholic beverages contain carbohydrates and sugars. For example, most beer comes from malted cereal grains, most commonly malted barley and malted wheat.

<u>WHAT TO DRINK?</u>

Water, tea and coffee (decaffeinated) should be your beverages. In a restaurant setting, order water for your drink. Many people order a soda or a dessert in a restaurant under peer pressure. Remember your body has *not* changed because you are in a restaurant.

WHAT TO EAT?

1. Vegetables

For clarification, when I use the term vegetables, I refer to the leaf and stem part of the plant, excluding the roots (such as potatoes, sweet potatoes and yam), which are basically starches.

Eat plenty of vegetables. Include vegetables in every meal. They are a great source of vitamins, minerals and fiber. They are bulk forming, fill up your stomach and satisfy your appetite. They also *slow* down the absorption of sugar from carbohydrates in your diet.

In general, vegetables contain only small amounts of carbohydrates, which is usually fiber. For example, 1/2 cup of cooked spinach contains only 3 gm of carbohydrates, out of which 2 gm is fiber. Spinach, like many other green leafy vegetables, is a great source of Vitamin A, Vitamin K and Manganese.

Use fresh vegetables of the season. Get them from your own vegetable garden or from a farmers' market. Try to steam them or lightly fry in olive oil.

Use raw vegetables in your salads, such as cucumber, bell pepper, spinach and tomatoes.

Certain vegetables are particularly good for patients with Graves' disease. Why? Because these vegetables may *decrease* the synthesis of thyroid hormone in the thyroid gland.

These vegetables are:

Cauliflower, Cabbage, Broccoli, Spinach, Bamboo Shoots, Bok Choy, Brussels Sprouts, Collard Greens and Kale.

Caution:

Avoid these vegetables if you become hypothyroid, as some patients with Graves' disease do in a matter of time, due to the progression of the autoimmune process.

2. Fruits

Eat one to two fresh fruits or 1/2 cup per day. Always use fruits which are in season. Either get them from your own fruit trees or from a farmers' market. Avoid fruits and vegetables which have traveled all around the world.

There is tremendous wisdom why certain fruits and vegetables grow in a certain season and climate. We humans may never be able to comprehend this wisdom. Suffice it is to say that if you *live in sync with nature*, you will avoid a lot of health problems.

For example, nature produces <u>summer</u> fruits for people in a particular area who are also experiencing <u>summer</u> temperatures. Now, you may be in the winter season, but your grocery store is loaded with summer fruits, brought thousand of miles away from the other side of the equator. Without thinking, you grab these produce items as novelty items. Remember fruits and vegetables are just foods, *not* items for mental entertainment or ego enhancement.

<u>Certain fruits are particularly good for patients with Graves' disease, as they contain chemicals which can decrease the synthesis of thyroid hormone. These fruits are Strawberries, Pears and Peaches.</u>

In general, fruits are a great source of vitamins and minerals, especially potassium. Fruits contain carbohydrates, but they are mainly simple sugars, *fructose*, which are easily absorbed from the intestines, because they do not require any further breakdown.

Fruits are a great source of antioxidants. In this way, they help to neutralize the damaging effects of <u>free oxygen radicals</u> that are released as a byproduct of the metabolism of food in the cell or when the body is exposed to cigarette smoking or radiation. These free oxygen radicals can damage the structures inside the cell. This is called <u>oxidative stress</u> and it may play a significant role in causing diseases such as cancer and heart disease. Anti-oxidants help to neutralize oxidative stress. Anti-oxidants consists of Beta-carotene, Vitamin A, Vitamin C, Vitamin E, Lutein, Lycopene and Selenium.

Brightly colored fruits are loaded with anti-oxidants. Fruits that are highest in antioxidant contents are pomegranate, blueberries, strawberries, cranberries, cherries, dates, plums, oranges, apples and pineapples.

Fruits are also a good source of fiber, especially avocados, apple, pear, guava, dates, cherimoya, pomegranate, passion fruit, blueberries, blackberries, raspberries, mango, orange, figs and kiwi fruit.

Avocado, guava, dates and cherimoya are a great source of protein. Avocados are also loaded with omega 3 fatty acids, vitamins C and E, carotenoids, selenium, zinc and phytosterols, which help to protect against heart disease and inflammation.

3. Nuts/Seeds

Nuts and seeds are an excellent source of nutrition. They are a great source of Monounsaturated Fatty Acids (MUFA) and omega-3 polyunsaturated fatty acids. Together, these are called the *good* fats. Why? Because these fats help to increase good (HDL) cholesterol and lower bad (LDL) cholesterol.

Nuts are also a good source of protein, vitamin E (an anti-oxidant) and fiber. They are also low in terms of carbohydrates. For example, 100 gm of almonds provides you with 21 grams of protein, 12 grams of fiber and only 20 grams of carbohydrates. Compare it to 100 grams of Quinoa, which provides you with roughly 13 grams of protein, 6 grams of fiber and 69 grams of carbohydrates.

Nuts are also packed with vitamins and minerals such as magnesium, phosphorus, potassium, selenium, manganese, folate, copper, calcium and zinc. In addition, nuts contain phytosterols, such as flavonoids, proanthocyanidins and phenolic acids.

There is mounting evidence to show that nuts may reduce oxidative stress and inflammation. Clinical studies show that nuts can reduce the risk of heart disease, age-related brain dysfunction and diabetes (1, 2).

Almonds, pine-nuts, pistachios and peanuts contain more protein than other nuts. Macadamias contains the highest amount of monounsaturated fatty acids, followed by hazelnuts, pecans, almonds, cashews, pistachios and Brazil nuts. Walnuts contain the highest amount of polyunsaturated fatty acids, followed by Brazil nuts, pecans, pine nuts, pistachios, peanuts, almonds and cashews.

Nuts also contain a small amount of saturated fat, the so called bad fat. <u>Almonds contain the least amount of saturated fat</u> and Brazil nuts the highest. <u>While all nuts contain some selenium, Brazil nuts have the highest quantities</u>. Selenium is a good antioxidant, helps the immune system and may prevent some cancers.

Pine nuts are one of the richest sources of <u>manganese</u>, which is an important co-factor for the <u>anti-oxidant</u> enzyme, superoxide dismutase. Consequently, pine nuts are good anti-oxidants. In addition, pine nuts contain the essential fatty acid <u>pinolenic acid,</u> which works as an <u>appetite-suppressant</u> by triggering the hunger suppressant enzymes, *cholecystokinin* and *glucagon-like peptide-1* (GLP-1) in the small intestine.

Technically, peanuts are not actually nuts but legumes. Dry beans, peas and lentils are some other examples of legumes.

Like nuts, seeds are a good source of protein. For example, 100 grams of seeds will provide you with 30 grams of protein. Seeds are an excellent source of the amino acids tryptophan and glutamate. Tryptophan is converted into serotonin and niacin. Serotonin is an important regulator of our mood. Low serotonin can lead to depression. That's why many modern anti-depressant medications, such as Prozac, Zoloft, Paxil, Celexa and Lexapro act by increasing the level of serotonin in the brain. Glutamate is a precursor for the synthesis of γ-amino butyric acid (GABA), which is an anti-stress neurotransmitter in the brain and can help to reduce your anxiety.

Like nuts, seeds are also loaded with vitamins and minerals. Pumpkin seeds can block the action of an androgen, DHEA (Dehydroepi-androsterone). This may be helpful in preventing prostate and ovarian cancers.

With so many health benefits, I strongly recommend that my patients with Graves' disease load up on nuts and seeds. Eat a handful (about 1 ounce) of nuts before each meal.

Use raw nuts and seeds. Do not use salted, sugar-coated or chocolate-coated nuts or seeds for obvious reasons.

4. Meats/Poultry/Fish

Eat meats, poultry and fish (fresh-water), including shell fish (farm-raised). Avoid fish and shell fish from the sea because it has high iodine content. Avoid processed meats, as these are loaded with preservatives and iodine.

Unprocessed meats are excellent sources of protein, vitamins, minerals and contain no carbohydrates. For example, 1 oz (28 grams) of cooked Atlantic salmon contains 6 grams of protein, 3 grams of fat, is loaded with Omega 3 fatty acids, and is also a good source of Thiamin, Niacin, Vitamin B6, Phosphorus, Vitamin B12 and Selenium (3).

Red meat is an excellent source of protein, iron and vitamins, especially vitamin B12. For example, 1 oz (28 grams) of ground Beef, (95% lean meat/5% fat, crumbles, cooked, pan-browned, hamburger) contains 8 grams of protein, 2 grams of fat, and No carbohydrates or sugar. It does contain 20 mg of cholesterol which is only 7% of the daily recommended value (4). Compare it to 1oz (28 grams) of cooked Quinoa which contains only 1 gram of protein, 1 gram of fat and 6 grams of carbohydrates, but no cholesterol (5).

Eat red meat 2 - 3 times per week. Select lean cuts. Avoid processed meats such as cold cuts, salami and hot dogs, as these often contain added sugar and carbohydrates.

Eat Chicken and/or turkey once a day. These are great sources of protein and vitamins.

Eat fresh-water fish 1 - 2 times a week. In addition to providing you with protein and vitamins, these are great source of Omega-3 fatty acids, which are good for your cardiovascular health. However, overconsumption of fish can lead to mercury poisoning. Avoid sea fish, which is high in iodine. For the same reason, avoid shell fish from the sea, but you can use farm-raised fish and shell fish.

Remember, vitamin B12 is lacking in plants. Therefore, you often become low in vitamin B12 if you are on a vegan OR vegetarian diet.

5. Dairy

Eat a cup of regular, plain yogurt everyday. It is a great source of healthy bacteria for our intestinal health. It is also a good source of protein and calcium as well.

Include a moderate amount of cheeses in your diet. If you are trying to lose weight, then limit the use of cheese.

Milk does contain significant amounts of iodine. Therefore, do not consume too much of milk. Moderation is the key. Drink a cup of milk per day, provided you are not Lactose Intolerant, which is more prevalent in patients with Graves' disease. If you have Lactose intolerance, you should try Almond milk. A lot of individuals with lactose intolerance do well on yogurt and cheeses.

6. Eggs

Eggs are a great source of protein, vitamins and minerals, especially Riboflavin, Vitamin B12, Phosphorus and Selenium. Eggs contain no carbohydrates. Therefore, they are a great nutritional source for people with Graves' disease.

However, avoid egg yolk, which is high in iodine. Also, cholesterol is present in the *yolk* of the egg. For these reasons, you should use only egg whites.

HOW TO EAT

Eat three regular meals per day. Dinner should be the lightest meal of the day, lunch the heaviest and breakfast the modest meal. Eat dinner at least 3 hours before bedtime.

Avoid snacks, especially when you're watching TV or working on a computer. If you absolutely must have a snack, then try something like nuts, carrot sticks or other raw vegetables.

Get involved in your food. Read labels on food while you are in the grocery store. You'll be surprised how many food items contain sugar, fructose syrup and corn syrup. Avoid these food items.

Try to prepare your meal yourself, at least over the weekend. Avoid buffets! When you opt for a buffet meal, you want to get the most for your buck (after all, you're only human) and you generally end up overeating. Try to eat at home as much as possible. You can find my original recipes in <u>Part 2</u> of this book.

If you are trying to lose weight, keep a diary of the food you eat. You may be amazed at how much you really eat, contrary to what you thought.

Eat when you are hungry, not because you're sad or on a computer or you have to socialize with family members and friends. People often eat because of psycho-social reasons. That's why they continue to gain weight.

Be aware of your eating habits. Eat slowly and enjoy every bite of your meal. Don't watch TV while eating. Many people overeat because they get too involved in watching a TV show or reading a newspaper and don't keep track of their food intake.

Read these recommendations frequently. This will serve as a reminder. Watch your conditioned mind and see how it tries to *lure* you to eat foods that you know you should not eat. Be aware of the inner voice such as, "Reward yourself. You deserve this bowl of ice-cream. Eat whatever because you're at a party." The inner voice comes from your conditioned mind, which is the basis of your old, bad, illogical eating behavior. You need to rise above it, simply by observing the inner voice, which actually is your enemy in the sense that it sabotages your health.

Practical suggestions for meals

<u>Breakfast:</u>

Egg white omelet using 2-3 egg whites only.

OR

2-4 hard boiled eggs (egg whites only).

1/2 to 1 cup of yogurt.

Lunch / Dinner:

A bowl of vegetable soup.

A plate of grilled chicken and fresh garden salad (you may add salad dressing).

A fresh fruit such as a small apple, pear, plum or a few strawberries.

OR

A bowl of vegetable soup.

A small chicken or turkey or tuna lettuce wrap.

A fresh fruit such as a small apple, pear, plum or a few strawberries.

OR

Grilled vegetables such as bell pepper, zucchini or eggplant with chicken or turkey strips stir fried.

A fresh fruit such as a small apple, pear, plum or a few strawberries.

OR

Steamed vegetables such as broccoli or cauliflower.

Grilled Chicken or Steak.

A small baked potato (without butter or sour cream).

A fresh fruit such as a small apple, pear, plum or a few strawberries.

OR

Shrimp (farm-raised) with vegetables on a small bed of pasta.

A fresh fruit such as a small apple, pear, plum or a few strawberries.

OR

A bowl of soup.

Fish (river), grilled or baked

A fresh fruit such as a small apple, pear, plum or a few strawberries.

Ethnic foods

Chinese

Beef or chicken or shrimp, cooked any Chinese style.

A fresh fruit such as a small apple, pear, plum or a few strawberries.

OR

Mongolian barbeque beef or chicken.

A fresh fruit such as a small apple, pear, plum or a few strawberries.

Japanese

Avoid rice rolls.

Stir fried beef or chicken.

A fresh fruit such as a small apple, pear, plum or a few strawberries.

Mexican

A cup of vegetable soup.

 A plate of chicken or beef fajitas, without tortillas.

A fresh fruit such as a small apple, pear, plum or a few strawberries.

Indian/ Pakistani

Two pieces of Tandoori chicken.

Mixed vegetables.

A fresh fruit such as a small apple, pear, plum or a few strawberries.

OR

Two Seekh Kebobs.

A plate of vegetables such as okra, spinach, cauliflower or eggplant.

A fresh fruit such as a small apple, pear, plum or a few strawberries.

OR

A small portion of chicken or beef or lamb curry, mixed with vegetables. For example, lamb saag or lamb okra or chicken jalfrezi.

A fresh fruit such as a small apple, pear, plum or a few strawberries.

Middle East

Chicken or beef kebob and salad.

A fresh fruit such as a small apple, pear, plum or a few strawberries.

OR

Chicken shawarma.

Grilled vegetables.

A fresh fruit such as a small apple, pear, plum or a few strawberries.

Greek

Greek salad.

Gyro meat (no fries or rice).

A fresh fruit such as a small apple, pear, plum or a few strawberries.

Please refer to PART 2 of the book for RECIPES

References:

1. O'Neil, C.E., D.R. Keast, T.A. Nicklas, V.L. Fulgoni, 2011. Nut consumption is associated with decreased health risk factors for cardiovascular disease and metabolic syndrome in U.S. adults: NHANES 1999–2004. Journal of the American College of Nutrition. 30(6):502–510.

2. Carey, A.N., S.M. Poulose, B. Shukitt-Hale, 2012. The beneficial effects of tree nuts on the aging brain. *Nutrition and Aging*. 1:55–67. DOI 10.3233/NUA-2012-0007.

3. http://nutritiondata.self.com/facts/finfish-and-shellfish-products/4259/2

4. http://nutritiondata.self.com/facts/beef-products/6192/2

5. http://nutritiondata.self.com/facts/cereal-grains-and-pasta/10352/2

Chapter **12**

Vitamin D Supplementation

You may recall from Chapter 9 that Vitamin D plays an important role in the *normal* functioning of the immune system. There is strong scientific evidence to incriminate low vitamin D as an important factor in the causation of autoimmune diseases such as rheumatoid arthritis, lupus, fibromyalgia, multiple sclerosis and Type 1 diabetes. In an experimental study from UCLA School of Medicine, Vitamin D deficiency was found to cause Graves' disease.

My clinical experience at *the Jamila Diabetes and Endocrine Medical Center* shows Vitamin D to be low in every patient with autoimmune diseases, including patients with Graves' disease.

You may wonder, why do I need Vitamin D supplementation? I live in a sunny place, spend at least 15 minutes a day in the sun, drink milk and take a daily multivitamin, which contains 100% of the recommended dose of Vitamin D. Shouldn't I have enough Vitamin D?

An Epidemic Of Vitamin D Deficiency

Believe it or not, there's an epidemic of Vitamin D deficiency! Ten years ago, I started investigating Vitamin D levels in my patients. To my surprise, the vast majority turned out to be low in Vitamin D. My experience is in line with other researchers. For example, researchers recently analyzed the data on Vitamin D status in the U.S. adult population from the 2000-2004 National Health and Nutrition Examination Survey (NHANES) (1). They were amazed to discover that 50-78% of Americans were low in Vitamin D. What's alarming is that the situation is getting worse. Vitamin D levels in Americans were found to be lower during the 2000-2004 period compared to the 1988-1994 period (2). Clearly Vitamin D deficiency is getting out of control.

Not only Americans, but people all around the world are suffering from Vitamin D deficiency. For example, in the United Kingdom, 90% of adults were found to be low in Vitamin D according to the nationally representative data collected between 1992 and 2001 (3). Vitamin D deficiency is the true epidemic of our times. It is perhaps more common than any other medical condition at the present time.

It Spares No Age

Infants, children, adults and elderly are all low in Vitamin D. In my extensive clinical experience, it's rare to find someone who has a good level of Vitamin D. In my practice, the age of patients range from 15 to 95. I find an overwhelming majority of these patients to be low in Vitamin D. Several studies have clearly demonstrated that Vitamin D deficiency spans across all age groups.

It Spares No Geographic Location

According to an old paradigm, Vitamin D deficiency exists only in northern areas with severe prolonged winters such as Canada, the Northeastern U.S., the U.K. and other northern European countries. However, in reality, Vitamin D deficiency is prevalent even in sunny, warm places such as the Middle East, India, Pakistan, New Zealand and Australia. In my own extensive clinical experience in southern California, I have found that most of my patients are low in Vitamin D. Vitamin D deficiency is a global phenomenon.

If you live in northern climates, you are more prone to Vitamin D deficiency because you can't get enough Vitamin D during winter months. In places above 42 degrees North latitude (approximately a line drawn between the northern border of California and Boston), there isn't sufficient solar UVB (Ultra Violet B) energy to form Vitamin D in the skin during winter time (from November through February). In far northern latitudes, this decrease in solar energy may last up to 6 months.

In areas below 34 degrees North latitude (approximately a line drawn between Los Angeles and Columbia, North Carolina), there's enough solar UVB energy for skin synthesis of Vitamin D throughout the year. But even in these areas, the sun can't give you Vitamin D if you avoid it by using clothing, sun screen lotions or by simply staying out of it. Therefore, you may live in a sunny place south of 34 degrees latitude, but still be low in Vitamin D.

Several clinical studies have shown that Vitamin D deficiency is extremely common in the sunny Middle East, primarily because the skin doesn't get enough sun exposure. Due to cultural habits, people avoid the sun and cover most of their body with clothes. This is particularly true in the case of women living in these countries.

It Spares No Race

Although darker skin is less efficient in synthesizing Vitamin D from sun exposure as compared to fair skin, people with fair skin avoid the sun more than people with dark skin for fear of skin cancer. In my extensive clinical experience, I've found people from various racial and ethnic groups to be low in Vitamin D.

What Are The Causes For The Epidemic Of Vitamin D Deficiency?

1. Modern Life-Style

Let's take a historic look at Vitamin D. It appears that humans started their journey on planet Earth in Africa where there was plenty of sunshine. With slow migration northwards over thousands of years, the skin gradually adapted to colder northern climates by reducing the content of its natural sun screen (melanin) and consequently, skin became lighter in color. People with light skin were then able to synthesize enough Vitamin D in brief exposures to sunshine.

Vitamin D deficiency is a relatively new phenomenon. Scientists first recognized it in the seventeenth century in the U.K. and other Northern European countries. Interestingly, it coincided with the period of the Industrial Revolution when people flocked to big industrial cities such as London and Warsaw and lived in multistoried buildings with narrow, dark alleys. Pollution from coal burning factories created a thick layer of smog. These factors significantly reduced the amount of sun rays reaching Earth in these regions, which already had marginal sunshine during long winter periods.

The phenomenon of the Industrial Revolution continued in the newly discovered lands of America and Canada. In addition, native Africans were enslaved and transported in ships to America over a period of months. Compare this rapid migration to the thousands of years it took for early Africans to migrate to Europe, allowing for their skin to adapt to less sunshine. In contrast, this recent migration was extraordinarily rapid, allowing no time for the skin to adapt to conditions of less sunshine. For this reason, African-Americans as a group are particularly low in Vitamin D. In recent years, worldwide migration happens at an even faster pace. In a matter of hours, you can migrate from one region of the world to another. That's why people from India and Pakistan who migrate to the U.K and North America are particularly low in Vitamin D.

Now consider another interesting phenomenon. As a result of the Industrial Revolution, people with fair skin were able to rapidly migrate to Southern regions with plenty of sunshine. Their skin didn't have time to adapt to these new, sunny environments. Therefore, these fair skinned people started developing skin cancer from excessive sun exposure. This led to the development of sunscreen lotions and the drum beat of "avoid the sun!" Even people with dark skin started applying sunscreen lotion under the impression that "it's a healthy habit."

The main reason we're facing an epidemic of Vitamin D deficiency is our modern life-style, which minimizes our exposure to the sun. Our technological revolution has dramatically changed lifestyles around the globe. Most people work indoors. They leave their homes early in the morning and return home around sunset or even after dark (especially during winter time). Even at lunch, most people drive to a restaurant or stay inside to eat. Many people spend their lunch break in their office. Over the weekend, we watch TV or surf the internet for entertainment. Teenagers usually stay indoors hooked to a computer or playing video games rather than going outdoors and playing real sports. While shopping, people are mostly indoors thanks to huge grocery stores and shopping malls. Many of the elderly live in assisted living facilities or nursing homes and don't get any sun exposure. Just observe yourself. How often do you, your family and friends stay indoors while carrying out usual activities of daily living?

2. Sun Phobia

Over the last 30 years or so, sun avoidance has been successfully drilled into the minds of the general public. People are simply scared of the ill-effects of the sun, including skin cancer, wrinkles and aging spots. Due to sun phobia, people avoid sun exposure at all costs. When we go outside for even a little while, we make sure to apply sun screen. Parents compulsively apply sunscreen before they allow their children to go outdoors. Many people don't realize that sunscreen also prevents Vitamin D synthesis in the skin.

3. Obesity

Vitamin D is fat soluble. Therefore, it gets stored in the fat in your body. In obese individuals, there is excessive storage of Vitamin D in fat. Consequently, the circulating level of Vitamin D is low in these individuals. Obesity has reached epidemic proportions in the U.S. and the rest of the world is also catching up in this regard. The epidemic of obesity is contributing to the epidemic of Vitamin D deficiency. It's interesting to note that in most cases, obesity is a product of our modern life-style as well.

4. Medical Illnesses

A. Malabsorption

Because Vitamin D is fat soluble, Vitamin D deficiency can develop in medical conditions that cause malabsorption of fat, such as surgical resection of the small intestine and stomach, chronic pancreatitis, pancreatic surgery, celiac sprue, Crohn's colitis and cystic fibrosis.

B. Liver and Kidney Diseases

Vitamin D from the blood is taken up by the liver where it is transformed into 25 (OH) Vitamin D, which in the kidneys is further transformed into 1,25 (OH)$_2$ Vitamin D. Therefore, Vitamin D deficiency develops in chronic liver disease, such as cirrhosis and in chronic kidney disease.

5. Medications

Some medications can further decrease Vitamin D level. These medications include: Phenytoin (brand name Dilantin), Phenobarbital, Rifampin, Orlistat (brand names Xenical and Alli), Cholestyramine (brand names Questran, LoCholest and Prevalite) and Steroids.

I often see patients who have been on these drugs for a long time, yet they're completely unaware these drugs can rob them of Vitamin D. They react with disbelief when I inform them about the relationship between these medications and Vitamin D deficiency. "Why didn't my other doctor tell me about it?" is their usual question. Of course, it's your doctor's responsibility to inform you about the side-effects of medicines. Unfortunately, the reality is that some do and some don't. So educate yourself and be a partner in taking charge of your health. That's why you're reading this book. Nothing can be more rewarding for me than providing you with the information you need to help take care of your Vitamin D needs in collaboration with your health care provider.

6. Flaws With The Current Recommendations On Vitamin D Intake

Many people taking vitamins assume that their Vitamin D level is okay because the label on their vitamin bottle says it meets 100% of the daily requirements. This misconception is one of the major reasons for Vitamin D deficiency among those people who are proactive in taking care of their health. Vitamin manufacturers follow government guidelines for the daily recommended amounts of various vitamins and minerals. Currently, the recommended daily allowance of Vitamin D in the U.S. is: 600 I.U. (International Units) from birth to age 70 and 800 I.U. if you are older than 70.

Most researchers in the field of Vitamin D (myself included) find these recommendations for Vitamin D to be inadequate. In a review article published in the July 2006 issue of the *American Journal of Clinical Nutrition*, the authors concluded that for most people, the optimal level of Vitamin D is not attainable with the current recommended daily allowances of Vitamin D (4). In March 2007, a number of researchers published an editorial urging a change in the recommendations on daily intake of Vitamin D to 1700 I.U in order to obtain a desirable blood level of Vitamin D (5).

DIAGNOSIS OF VITAMIN D DEFICIENCY

It's easy to diagnose Vitamin D deficiency: It's a simple blood test. That's all! However, it needs to be the right test and must be interpreted properly! And that's where a lot of problems arise.

What's The Right Test To Diagnose Vitamin D Deficiency And Why?

Laboratories offer two tests to determine Vitamin D level in the blood. In Vitamin D deficiency, one of them is low whereas the other one is often normal. Most physicians don't know the distinction between these two tests and may order the wrong test. Consequently, they may say your Vitamin D level is normal, when it's actually low.

The Correct Blood Test To Evaluate Your Vitamin D Status Is: <u>25 (OH) Vitamin D (25-Hydroxy Vitamin D).</u>
The other blood test for Vitamin D is $1,25 (OH)_2$ vitamin D (1,25 dihydroxy vitamin D). *This is the wrong test to diagnose Vitamin D deficiency! Why?*

There are two reasons why 25 (OH) vitamin D and not $1,25 (OH)_2$ vitamin D is the right test to diagnose Vitamin D deficiency.

Reason 1

25 (OH) vitamin D stays in your blood for a much longer period of time (half life of about 3 weeks) compared to $1,25 (OH)_2$ vitamin D (half life of about 14 hours). Therefore, 25 (OH) vitamin D more accurately reflects the status of Vitamin D in your body.

Reason 2

As Vitamin D deficiency develops, your body increases the production of parathyroid hormone by the parathyroid glands situated in your neck. Parathyroid hormone increases the conversion of 25 (OH) vitamin D into 1,25 $(OH)_2$ vitamin D. Consequently, 1,25 $(OH)_2$ vitamin D level in the blood will stay in the normal range (and can even be high) even if you're low in 25 (OH) vitamin D.

Why Are The Normal Ranges For 25 (OH) Vitamin D Inaccurate?

The normal ranges for Vitamin D come from the era when our concern was just to prevent rickets. A small dose of Vitamin D is enough to prevent rickets. Therefore, a level of 25 (OH) vitamin D of 10 ng/ml (25 nmol/L) or above was established as adequate to prevent rickets. That's why many laboratories report 10 ng/ml (25 nmol/L) as the lower limit of the normal range.

However, in recent years our understanding of the effects of Vitamin D has dramatically changed. Now we understand that Vitamin D can do much more than simply prevent rickets. In fact, Vitamin D is crucial for maintaining many vital functions in the body, such as a healthy immune system and a healthy heart. In addition, an adequate level of Vitamin D helps prevent diabetes, osteoporosis and cancer.

To achieve these goals, many experts in the field (myself included) recommend a level of 25 (OH) vitamin D to be at least 30 ng/ml (75 nmol/L) and preferably above 50 ng/ml (125 nmol/L). An excellent review of scientific studies (4) published in the *American Journal of Clinical Nutrition* in 2006 concluded that the most beneficial blood level of 25 (OH) vitamin D starts at 30 ng/ml (or 75 nmol/L).

Unfortunately, many laboratories continue to report a normal range with the lower limit of 10 ng/ml (25 nmol/L). Now imagine the following scenario: Your 25 (OH) vitamin D level is 19 ng/ml.; Your physician interprets this as normal because it's in the "normal range" provided by the laboratory. However, you are actually quite low in Vitamin D! This happens all too frequently.

Watch Out For The Units Used By The Laboratory

There is another problem that many physicians are unaware of. Different laboratories report Vitamin D level in different units. In the U.S. and around the world, most laboratories report 25 (OH) vitamin D in one of two ways: either as ng/ml or nmol/L.

The conversion factor from ng/ml to nmol/L is about 2.5. For example, if your level is 30 ng/ml, you multiply it by 2.5 and you will get a number of 75 in nmol/L. The lower limit of normal for 25 (OH) vitamin D should be 30 ng/ml or 75 nmol/L.

Now, let's assume that you are fortunate enough to have a physician who keeps up with the latest information and is proactive about Vitamin D supplementation. From attending conferences and reading articles on Vitamin D, your physician may simply remember that the lower limit of normal for 25 (OH) vitamin D is 30 (and that's how most physicians remember - just the numbers, without paying attention to the units).

Here's another treacherous case scenario: Your laboratory reports your 25 (OH) vitamin D to be 40 nmol/L. Your physician simply looks at the number 40 and tells you your Vitamin D is good. In his mind, it's more than 30, so you're fine. In fact, your Vitamin D is low because in reality, a level of 40 nmol/L is equal to 16 ng/ml.!! He totally *forgot* to look closely at the units.

Also, note that the upper limit of normal as reported by many laboratories is also inaccurate. The upper limit of normal should be 100 ng/ml (250 nmol/L).

TREATMENT OF VITAMIN D DEFICIENCY

Most physicians do not know how to properly treat Vitamin D deficiency. Why? Because it's not taught during their medical training, nor do they have much experience in their clinical practice. It's a new field for them.

What amazes me is the advice given in newspaper articles, such as "experts recommend that either 600 units of Vitamin D a day or 15 minutes of sunshine a day is enough to get a good level of Vitamin D." I believe these recommendations are flawed.

Why is the Recommended Daily Dose Of Vitamin D Inaccurate?

I check Vitamin D level in all of my patients. The majority turn out to be low in Vitamin D. Many of them take the recommended dose of 600 I.U. of Vitamin D a day. Many of them also go out in the sun at least 15 minutes a day in sunny southern California, yet they're still low in Vitamin D. Based on this kind of sound clinical evidence, it's clear to me that 600 I.U. of Vitamin D a day is insufficient. Fifteen minutes of sunshine a day is also insufficient to get a good level of Vitamin D.

It's also unscientific to make general recommendations about how much sun exposure can provide you with enough Vitamin D. Why? There are many variables that determine Vitamin D level in your body including:

1. Latitude

In areas north of 44 degrees N latitude, sun rays are less effective in producing Vitamin D in the skin during winter months. The farther north you live, the less effective skin synthesis is from sun exposure.

2. Season

In the same region, the sun is less intense during winter months. Consequently, skin synthesis of Vitamin D decreases during wintertime.

3. Age

As you grow older, the skin becomes less efficient in synthesizing Vitamin D from sun exposure.

4. Skin Color

The darker your skin, the less efficient it is in forming Vitamin D from sun exposure.

5. Sun screens

If you use sunscreen, then your skin can't form Vitamin D even if you live in a sunny area like Los Angeles or Miami.

6. Lifestyle

Obviously, if you stay out of the sun, you can't form Vitamin D in your skin. Many people work indoors and choose leisure activities that are indoors. Similarly, if you cover your entire skin due to cultural reasons (like many women in the Middle-East), you can't form Vitamin D from your skin, even though you live in a sunny place.

Use logic and see for yourself. With so many variables determining Vitamin D level, how could "spending 15 minutes a day in the sun" be an accurate recommendation? For example, a New Yorker spending 15 minutes a day in the sun will have a different Vitamin D level than a Texan. Even in New York, a person with fair skin will have a different Vitamin D level than a person with dark skin. A teenager will have a different level than a grandparent. The same New Yorker will have a different level of Vitamin D during summer versus winter. You can see why the "15 minutes of sunshine a day recommendation" is flawed. The "one size fits all" approach doesn't work with an issue that has so many variables!

My Approach To the Treatment Of Vitamin D Deficiency

Over the last fifteen years, I've treated thousands of patients with Vitamin D deficiency. Based on my own clinical observations, I've developed a unique, scientific yet practical treatment approach that works well for my patients.

1. Assess Vitamin D Status

First of all, I assess and treat every person on an individual basis. I order a 25 (OH) vitamin D level in the blood to assess Vitamin D status. This accurately reflects the impact of variables in lifestyle such as geographic location, season, ethnicity, working habits, eating habits, outdoor activities and sunscreen application habits. No guess work. No blind recommendations. To me, this is the most scientific approach in determining one's Vitamin D status!

2. Aim For An Optimal Level Of Vitamin D

After the lab test, I discuss the results with my patients. As I wrote earlier, the level of 25 (OH) vitamin D should be at least 30 ng/ml (75 nmol/L). Now you may ask, "But what is the optimal level of Vitamin D?" Based on my extensive experience, I believe <u>the optimal blood level of 25 (OH) vitamin D to be in the range of 50-100 ng/ml (125-250 nmol/L)</u>. I feel that a Vitamin D concentration at this level is important in order to normalize immune function, build strong bones, treat body aches and pains and prevent cancer, heart disease, osteoporosis, tooth fractures, diabetes, high blood pressure, kidney disease and depression.

3. How To Achieve A Good Level Of Vitamin D

I discuss with each individual patient how to achieve an optimal level of Vitamin D.

<u>You can get Vitamin D from Four Sources:</u>

> A. Sun exposure
> B. Diet
> C. Vitamin D supplements
> D. Ultraviolet lamps

For an average person, it's impossible to get a good level of Vitamin D from sun exposure or diet alone. For example, according to my experience, a Caucasian person needs to be out in the sun in southern California in a bathing suit for approximately two to four hours a day to get a good level of Vitamin D. Now how many people can have that kind of lifestyle year round?

In my extensive experience of diagnosing and treating Vitamin D deficiency, I encountered only one person with a good blood level of 25 (OH) vitamin D (above 50 ng/ml without taking any supplements). She was a lifeguard with fair skin who spent about four hours a day, five days a week in the sun in her bathing suit. This amount of sun exposure is not only impractical, but also inadvisable. This degree of sun exposure significantly increases your risk for skin cancer, especially if you have fair skin.

Now consider this: One 8 ounce cup of milk has only 100 I.U. of Vitamin D. You'd have to drink 40-60 cups a day to get a good level of Vitamin D. It's not only impractical, but also inadvisable. Imagine all the calories, the amount of LDL (bad) cholesterol and the natural sugar you'd get from such a huge amount of milk.

A serving of cereal fortified with Vitamin D has about 40-80 I.U. of Vitamin D. You can imagine how much cereal you'd have to eat to get a good level of vitamin D. There are many negative consequences to eating such a large amount of cereal.

From a practical stand point, I recommend taking advantage of three sources of Vitamin D: sun, diet and Vitamin D supplements. I never resort to ultraviolet lamps, which are expensive and in my experience, unnecessary.

THE THREE SOURCES OF VITAMIN D

1. Sun exposure

The Sun is an excellent source of Vitamin D, but it can also cause skin cancer. Various physicians make extreme recommendations on sun exposure, depending upon their specialty. Dermatologists, with their tunnel vision, exaggerate the fear of skin cancer and recommend avoiding the sun as much as possible... And don't forget to put on sunscreen each time you go outside! On the other hand, physicians solely interested in vitamin D, with their tunnel vision, recommend liberal sun exposure and minimize the fear of skin cancer. In my opinion, both have myopic views, which unfortunately is a basic flaw inherent to modern medicine. Physicians think in the narrow range of their own specialty and don't consider the overall, whole outlook for the patient.

My Recommendations About Sun Exposure

Living in the modern world, you can't obtain a good level of Vitamin D simply from sun exposure. However, you should try to get some of your Vitamin D from the sun.

Here's my sensible approach to sun exposure:

- People with dark skin, without any history of skin cancer, should spend about 60 minutes a day in the sun, without any sunscreen, between 10 am and 3 pm. If weather permits, try not to cover your arms or your legs below the knees.

- People with fair skin, without any history of skin cancer, should go out in the sun for short periods, about 10 -15 minutes a day, without any sunscreen, between 10 am and 3 pm.

- The duration of sun exposure can be a bit more during winter months and a little less during summer months.

- People with a history of skin cancer should avoid the sun as much as possible and wear sunscreen when they are outdoors.

2. Diet

Diet is not a good source of Vitamin D. However, you can get some Vitamin D from diet. Please note that when you select food, Vitamin D should not be the only consideration. You need to take a more comprehensive approach when selecting food, paying attention to overall ingredients.

Different people have different nutritional requirements, depending on numerous factors such as age, genetics, weight, metabolism, physical activity, seasonal variation and medical conditions such as diabetes, cholesterol disorder, high blood pressure, heart disease, metabolic syndrome, menopause symptoms, polycystic ovary syndrome, thyroid disorders and other medical conditions.

As I mentioned earlier, modern medicine suffers from "narrow-mindedness" in the sense that every expert gives advice according to his/her specialty without looking at the overall person as a whole. That's why there are so many different diets, each conflicting with the other, each claiming to be better than the other.

Consider this scenario: In a magazine article, an expert recommends drinking plenty of orange juice, because it contains 100 I.U. of Vitamin D per cup. So you start drinking a lot of orange juice without realizing that you're also consuming large quantities of sugar and potassium in the orange juice. If you happen to be diabetic, your glucose values will go through the roof. If you have Metabolic Syndrome and are pre-diabetic, your insulin level will skyrocket. If you're an elderly person with diabetes, high blood pressure and kidney failure, your blood sugar will shoot up and your blood potassium may also become elevated, which if not diagnosed and treated appropriately, can be life threatening. As you can see, you can get in a real mess just because you were myopically focusing on improving your Vitamin D level.

So, please beware of all ingredients in a food, not just its Vitamin D content.

With this understanding, let us take a closer look at some foods and their Vitamin D contents:

MILK
    Natural milk does not contain Vitamin D, but milk in the U.S. and many other countries is fortified with Vitamin D. However, even fortified milk contains only 100 I.U. per cup (8 oz or 240 ml).

Drink one to two cups a day. In this way, you get about 100-200 I.U. of Vitamin D and other components of milk in a small to moderate amount. Milk is a good source of calcium. It's also a good source of protein and also contains some natural sugar and some fat.

Milk is a much better choice than soft drinks, which are loaded with sugar or other artificial sweeteners, which can have a lot of side-effects. Diet drinks have no real nutritional value. Another disadvantage: soft drinks don't have any Vitamin D. People with lactose intolerance obviously should either drink Lactose free milk or avoid milk altogether.

YOGURT

Some yogurts have added Vitamin D. Yogurt is also an excellent source of calcium as well as Lactobacillus, friendly bacteria, which is very important for the health of your intestines.

CHEESE

Some cheeses contain a small amount of Vitamin D. Cheeses are fattening and are also loaded with iodine and LDL (bad) cholesterol. For these reasons, I advise patients to limit the amount of cheeses in their diet.

FISH

Oily fish such as salmon, mackerel and blue fish naturally contain reasonable amounts of Vitamin D. The amount of Vitamin D in fish remains unchanged if it is baked, but decreases about 50% if the fish is fried. Also, farm raised salmon has only about 25% of Vitamin D as compared to wild salmon.

A word of caution about fish consumption!

Fish from the sea is high in iodine content. Therefore, patients with Graves' disease should avoid sea fish. Too much fish consumption can also lead to mercury poisoning.

Fish with high mercury content include shark, whale, swordfish, king mackerel, tilefish and tuna (both fresh and frozen tuna). However, canned tuna doesn't seem to be high in mercury because it consists of smaller, shorter-lived species. But canned tuna does contain high amounts of iodine, and should be avoided by patients with Graves' disease.

Fresh water fish which can be high in mercury include bass, pike, and muskellunge.

Therefore, I recommend caution when consuming fish. Moderation is the key. Avoid those fish that contain high levels of mercury and iodine. This is particularly true for pregnant women, lactating women, young children and women of child bearing age, as the developing brain of the fetus and newborn is very susceptible to the injurious effects of mercury. For this reason, the Food and Drug Administration recommends that pregnant women, breast feeding women and young children should avoid eating fish with high mercury content.

Other food items

Other foods that contain very small amounts of Vitamin D include vegetables, meats and egg yolk.
The following food items are supposed to contain the indicated amount of Vitamin D.

Food	Serving Size	Vitamin D Content
Salmon, cooked	3.5 ounces	360, I.U.
Mackerel, cooked	3.5 ounces	345, I.U.
Canned Tuna	3.0 ounces	200, I.U.
Sardines canned in oil	1.75 ounces	250, I.U.
Raw shiitake mushroom	10 ounces	76, I.U.
Fortified milk	8 oz/240 ml	100, I.U.
Fortified orange juice	8 oz/240 ml	100, I.U.
Fortified cereal	1 serving	40-80, I.U.
Egg, (vitamin D is in yolk)	1 whole	20, I.U.
Liver of beef, cooked	3.5 oz	15, I.U.
Swiss cheese	1 oz	12, I.U.

I.U. = International Units

In the U.S., most cereals and orange juices are fortified with small amounts of Vitamin D.

A Word of Caution!

You can't simply rely on the stated quantities of Vitamin D in a food item. For example, in one study, researchers found that Vitamin D in milk was less than 80% of the stated amount (6). Also, Vitamin D content of fish is highly variable.

3. Vitamin D Supplements

From a practical perspective, you don't get enough Vitamin D from sun exposure and food. As I mentioned earlier, in my clinical practice in Southern California, I have encountered only one young lady who had a good level of Vitamin D from sun exposure alone, without any Vitamin D supplement. She was a life guard at the beach. For the rest of us, Vitamin D supplements become the major source of Vitamin D.

The Starting Dose Of Vitamin D Supplement

The starting dose of Vitamin D supplement varies from person to person. It mainly depends on how low your Vitamin D level is. So please get your 25 (OH) Vitamin D level checked and then use the following table as a guide to choose the starting dose of Vitamin D3.

Table To Calculate The Starting Dose Of Vitamin D Supplement

25 (OH) Vitamin D level in ng/ml	Dose of Vitamin D3
Less than 30	15,000 I.U. a day
30 - 40	10,000 I.U. a day
41 - 50	5,000 I.U. a day

Your Vitamin D dose also depends upon your body weight. The heavier you are, the more Vitamin D you need. Why? Because Vitamin D is *fat soluble* and gets trapped in fat. For this reason, obese people require a larger dose compared to thin people.

The above recommendations are for an average adult, with a weight of about **150 Lbs.**

As a guide, add 1000 I.U. for each 10 Lbs. above 150 Lbs. And subtract 1000 I.U. for each 10 lbs. below 150 Lbs.

Pay Attention To The Units On Your Vitamin D Supplement!

In the U.S., the dose of Vitamin D is available in I.U. However, in some parts of the world, Vitamin D is available in microgram (mcg).

Here is the conversion factor:
40 I.U. = 1 mcg

For example:
    600 I.U. = 15 mcg
    1,000 I.U. = 25 mcg
    5,000 I.U. = 125 mcg
    50,000 I.U. = 1250 mcg or 1.25 mg

VITAMIN D2, 50,000 I.U.

When Vitamin D level is below 20, an alternative treatment is to take a high dose of Vitamin D2. This is usually given as 50,000 I.U. per week for about 12 weeks. In the U.S., you need a physician's prescription for this dose of Vitamin D2.

Recently, Vitamin D3 also became available in a dose of 50,000 I.U., which is preferred over Vitamin D2.

The Maintenance Dose Of Vitamin D Supplement

A common problem arises from traditional medical training which teaches that once your Vitamin D stores are replenished, you go back to a daily maintenance dose of 600 I.U. a day. For example, if your Vitamin D is very low (let's say less than 15 ng/ml), your physician will likely place you on a high dose of Vitamin D2 such as 50,000 I.U a week for 12 weeks and afterwards, put you back on 600 I.U a day as a maintenance dose.

Most likely, in the following months, your physician won't check to see what happens to your Vitamin D level on this miniscule dose. This kind of practice is based on the medical myth hammered into physicians that once you've replenished Vitamin D stores, the problem is somehow cured.

Take a closer look at this myth. Vitamin D stays in your body stores for just a few weeks. Therefore, the "so called cure" of low Vitamin D will only last a few weeks and then you'll be back to your usual state of a low level of Vitamin D.

For this reason, I check Vitamin D level in my patients every three months. What I've discovered is eye opening! In my clinical experience, the maintenance dose of Vitamin D depends on the initial starting dose. For example, if a patient requires a high initial starting dose, that patient will need a high maintenance dose. Most people continue to require a high dose of Vitamin D to maintain a good level. It makes perfect sense. Why?

It's the overall lifestyle of a person that determines the level of Vitamin D. If a person is very low in Vitamin D to begin with, it's due to life-style, which in most cases doesn't change after a few weeks of Vitamin D therapy. Therefore, it's important to continue a relatively high dose of Vitamin D as a maintenance dose, especially in those individuals who are very low in Vitamin D to start with.

Most of my patients require a daily dose of 5,000 - 10,000 I.U. of Vitamin D3 to maintain a good level of Vitamin D. Some, especially obese individuals, need up to 20,000-25,000 I.U. a day, while some skinny individuals require only 2000 I.U. per day.

What Type Of Vitamin D?   D3 or D2?

Vitamin D2, also known as *ergocalciferol,* is of plant origin. On the other hand, Vitamin D3, also known as *cholecalciferol*, is of animal origin. In the natural state, humans synthesize Vitamin D3 in their skin upon exposure to sun. Therefore, I recommend Vitamin D3, as this is the physiological type of Vitamin D for humans.

Vitamin D: Oral (Swallowing) Or Sublingual (Under The Tongue)

I recommend the SUBLINGUAL (under the tongue) route for the absorption of Vitamin D supplement as compared to oral ingestion (swallowing). Why? Because sublingual absorption takes Vitamin D directly into general circulation, (medically known as *systemic circulation*), just like when Vitamin D is naturally synthesized in the skin from exposure to the sun.

In contrast, Vitamin D from oral ingestion is absorbed into local circulation (medically known as *portal circulation*) from the gut, which takes it to the liver first before entering into *systemic* circulation. In this way, oral ingestion is not very physiological and sublingual absorption is more physiological.

This point becomes even more important in people who have problems with digestion, such as people with pancreatitis, Crohn's disease, irritable bowel syndrome, gluten sensitivity, celiac disease and tropical sprue. It's also a problem for people who take medications that can interfere with the intestinal absorption of Vitamin D, such as seizure medicines, cholestyramine, orlistat and also for people with stomach bypass surgery, including those with lap-band procedures.

You can get Sublingual Vitamin D3 from online retailers. One such retailer's address is: http://powerofvitamind.com/sublingual_vitamin_d.html

Monitoring Vitamin D Level

I cannot *overemphasize* the need for close monitoring of your Vitamin D level. An individual's response to a dose of Vitamin D varies widely. As mentioned before, because Vitamin D is fat soluble, it gets trapped in fat. That means there is less Vitamin D available for the rest of the body. Therefore, obese people require a larger dose of Vitamin D than lean individuals. As Vitamin D is fat soluble, it requires normal intestinal mechanisms to absorb fat. If a person has some problem with fat absorption, such as patients with chronic pancreatitis, pancreatic surgery or stomach surgery, then they may *not* absorb Vitamin D adequately.

During summertime, the sun is stronger and many people spend time outdoors. Therefore, the required dose of Vitamin D supplement may go down a bit. In wintertime, the dose of Vitamin D may need to go up a bit. However, in a lot of individuals, this seasonal variation is minimal, because they mostly stay indoors and apply a good layer of sunscreen when they do go out. The amount of Vitamin D people get from their food also fluctuates considerably. In addition, some people take their Vitamin D supplement regularly, while others take it sporadically.

Therefore, I check 25 (OH) Vitamin D blood level every 3 months and adjust the dose of Vitamin D accordingly. My aim is to achieve and maintain a level of 25 (OH) Vitamin D in the range of 50-100 ng/ml.

I also check blood calcium to make sure that a person doesn't develop Vitamin D toxicity. I recommend monitoring Vitamin D and blood calcium level every three months. The blood test for calcium is part of a chemistry panel, usually referred to as CHEM 12 (chemistry 12) or CMP (Comprehensive Metabolic Panel). It's a routine blood test for most people who have an ongoing health issue such as diabetes, hypertension, cholesterol disorder, arthritis, etc.

Special Situations

1. STEROIDS

Because steroids interfere with your Vitamin D, I educate my patients to notify me if another doctor places them on a steroid.

When someone takes a high dose steroid in an oral form, such as Prednisone, or as an injection, such as Solumedrol, Depomedrol or Decadron, I *double* the dose of Vitamin D. I check their 25 (OH) Vitamin D level every 2 months and change the dose of Vitamin D accordingly.

2. CHILDREN AND TEENAGERS

Because human milk doesn't contain any appreciable amounts of Vitamin D, infants who are solely breastfed are at high risk for Vitamin D deficiency. Therefore, the American Academy of Pediatrics recently raised their recommended daily dose of Vitamin D to 400 I.U. in infants who are solely breastfed, beginning at the age of two months.

In most children, a daily dose of vitamin D3 of 1000 I.U. per 20 Lbs., seems appropriate. In addition, it makes sense to use sensible sun exposure, especially in infants and toddlers.

The teenage years are the time when most of your bone growth takes place. Therefore, teenagers need a good dose of Vitamin D and calcium. In my opinion, they should be encouraged to spend time outdoors and have sensible sun exposure. In addition, they should also take Vitamin D3 in a dose of 1000 I.U. per 20 Lbs.

3. PREGNANT AND BREASTFEEDING WOMEN

These women are at higher risk for Vitamin D deficiency. Low Vitamin D in the mother leads to low Vitamin D in the infant. Therefore, for pregnant and breastfeeding women, I check Vitamin D level at baseline and monitor it every two months. I treat their low Vitamin D as described earlier in this chapter.

If blood levels aren't available, then these women should take a dose of at least 5000 I.U. of Vitamin D3 a day.

4. MALABSORPTION SYNDROMES

Low Vitamin D is extremely common among people with malabsorption syndromes such as Crohn's disease, Celiac disease, chronic pancreatitis and intestinal, pancreatic or stomach surgeries.

In these patients, I check baseline Vitamin D level. I find that it is almost always very low. I treat low Vitamin D according to my strategy discussed earlier. These patients usually require a large dose of Vitamin D to meet their Vitamin D needs.

Now that Vitamin D3 is available in a SUBLINGUAL formulation, I strongly recommend it to these patients.

VITAMIN D TOXICITY

Every article written in newspapers and magazines about Vitamin D always includes an overly scary caution about Vitamin D toxicity. The reader gets the impression that it must be a common consequence of Vitamin D supplementation.

Some readers get so scared, they decide not to take Vitamin D supplementation and end up with the health consequences of Vitamin D deficiency. What a shame!

It's obvious to me that the writers of these magazine and newspaper articles don't actually treat patients with low Vitamin D and their knowledge about Vitamin D toxicity is very limited and superficial.

What Is Vitamin D Toxicity?

Vitamin D toxicity is defined as "too much Vitamin D, causing harm to the body."

What Level Of Vitamin D Causes Damage To The Body?

A blood level of 25 (OH) Vitamin D consistently more than 200 ng/ml (500 nmol/L) is considered to be potentially toxic (7). Please note "potentially toxic." It means that there is a potential risk for Vitamin D toxicity if your blood level is more than 200 ng/ml. However, it doesn't mean that you automatically suffer from Vitamin D toxicity if you're above 200 ng/ml. Indeed, in an animal model, blood concentration of Vitamin D up to 400 ng/ml (1000 nmol/L) was not associated with any toxicity (8).

The experts in the field of Vitamin D have chosen this cut off level of 200 ng/ml (500 nmol/L) arbitrarily in order to provide a safe limit. Please note that the normal range of 25 (OH) Vitamin D is 30-100 ng/ml (75-250 nmol/L).

How Frequent Is Vitamin D Toxicity?

Extremely rare.

I check Vitamin D level in all of my patients and been doing so over the last FIFTEEN years. *I haven't seen a single case of serious Vitamin D toxicity in my patients while they are on Vitamin D3 or D2 supplementation!* These patients are usually on a daily dose of 2,000 I.U. to 10,000 I.U. (50 mcg to 250 mcg) of Vitamin D3 or a weekly dose of Vitamin D2 of 50,000 I.U. (1.25 mg). None of these patients has had a level of 25 (OH) Vitamin D above 100 ng/ml (250 nmol/L).

Rarely, I see a patient with a slight increase in calcium level above the normal limit. Simply reducing calcium intake brings the calcium back into the normal range in these patients. I don't consider this slight increase in the calcium level as a case of Vitamin D toxicity. My experience is in line with other experts in the field of Vitamin D.

Over The Counter Vitamin D3 Versus Prescription Vitamin D, Calcitriol (Rocaltrol).

Let me clarify another issue. When medical writers of newspaper and magazine articles talk of Vitamin D toxicity, they make a blanket statement about Vitamin D supplements, which is a mistake. There are several different preparations of Vitamin D supplements. These include Vitamin D3 (cholecalciferol), Vitamin D2 (ergocalciferol), Calcidiol and Calcitriol. Calcitriol is also known as the brand name Rocaltrol.

Calcitriol (Rocaltrol) is a synthetic form of Vitamin D and is a drug rather than a supplement. Therefore, it requires a prescription from a physician. It is typically given to patients who have kidney failure and are on dialysis. Calcitriol (Rocaltrol) is also sometimes prescribed to patients whose parathyroid glands have been removed, often inadvertently by a surgeon during thyroid surgery. Calcitriol (Rocaltrol) is much more potent than natural Vitamin D3 or D2 and can sometimes result in Vitamin D toxicity. Physicians who prescribe calcitriol (Rocaltrol) are typically aware (and definitely should be aware) of this possibility and monitor their patients for Vitamin D toxicity.

Can You Develop Vitamin D Toxicity From Too Much Sun?

The answer is No. You can't develop Vitamin D toxicity from too much sun exposure. The reason? Nature is smart. The skin forms as much Vitamin D as the body needs. Beyond that, it degrades any excess Vitamin D that is formed in the skin (9). Pretty smart!

How Do You Detect Vitamin D Toxicity?

Vitamin D helps in the absorption of calcium from the intestines. Toxic levels of Vitamin D can cause an increase in blood level of calcium. Thus, Vitamin D toxicity manifests itself as a high level of calcium in the blood.

The simplest and the most scientific way to diagnose Vitamin D toxicity is to check your calcium and Vitamin D level in the blood. Everyone should have his/her Vitamin D level and calcium checked every three months. If your 25(OH) Vitamin D level is higher than 100 ng/ml (250 nmol/L) or your blood calcium gets elevated, then you should reduce your dose of Vitamin D. However, please note that you are still way below the potentially toxic level of 200 ng/ml (500 nmol/L).

Symptoms Of Vitamin D Toxicity

Symptoms of Vitamin D toxicity are due to increase in the blood level of calcium.

Mild increase in blood calcium level
Usually doesn't cause any symptoms.

Moderate increase in blood calcium
Usually causes non-specific symptoms of nausea, vomiting, constipation, poor appetite, weight loss and weakness. Remember these symptoms can be caused by a variety of other medical conditions as well.

Severe increase in blood calcium level

Causes neurologic symptoms such as somnolence, confusion, even coma and heart rhythm abnormalities, which can be fatal if not treated promptly.

Treatment OF Vitamin D Toxicity

Rarely, I see a patient whose blood calcium goes slightly above the upper limit of normal while on Vitamin D supplementation. I lower their calcium intake and repeat a blood test for calcium in a month. In my experience, the reduction in calcium intake brings down calcium into the normal range.

Very rarely, blood calcium remains slightly elevated. I then check parathyroid hormone level. If it is in the normal range, then I further discuss diet with the patient and try to lower calcium intake. Even in these very rare patients, blood calcium usually normalizes by lowering their calcium intake.

I also keep in mind other causes for elevated blood calcium level such as primary hyperparathyroidism and cancer. I order diagnostic testing in this regard on a case by case basis. If blood calcium is elevated and parathyroid hormone (PTH, intact) is also elevated and both of these values do not normalize with Vitamin D supplementation, then that patient is most likely suffering from primary hyperparathyroidism. If parathyroid hormone (PTH, intact) level is normal and the patient continues to have an elevated calcium level, I investigate the possibility of other causes of high calcium such as cancer.

Rarely, high blood calcium may occur due to Vitamin D toxicity, which can happen if very high doses of Vitamin D are used (such as 100,000 I.U. per day) for a long period. However, I have not seen it in my practice. In my experience, the usual doses of Vitamin D3 ranging from 5,000 I.U. to 10,000 I.U. per day do not cause high blood calcium.

Remember, there are many causes of an increase in blood calcium level other than Vitamin D toxicity. Two such common causes of high blood calcium are primary hyperparathyroidism and *cancer. If you have high blood calcium, your physician should thoroughly look into various causes of high blood calcium.*

It's important to notify your physician about all the dietary supplements, including Vitamin D, that you take. Most physicians don't specifically ask about dietary supplements and often patients don't think to provide this information either. For best medical care, your physician should know all the medicines, as well as all the dietary supplements, that you take. If your physician determines that a mild increase in your blood calcium level is due to excessive doses of "over the counter" Vitamin D supplementation, as evidenced by a high blood level of 25(OH) Vitamin D, in consultation with your physician, you should decrease the dose of your calcium intake and Vitamin D. In most cases, simply reducing the calcium intake will bring calcium back into the normal range. If your physician advises you to reduce the dose of Vitamin D, you should do so. Recheck your calcium level in a month or so to make sure that your blood calcium is back to normal. Recheck your Vitamin D and calcium in about 3 months to make sure that these levels are good and you haven't swung in the other direction.

If your blood calcium is high due to "prescription Vitamin D," such as calcitriol, the treatment will depend upon the degree of high blood calcium and your symptoms. Your physician will manage it accordingly. If your calcium level is moderate to severely high, your physician will likely admit you to the hospital for proper treatment of Vitamin D toxicity.

References:

1. Yetley EA, Assessing vitamin D status of the U.S. population. *Am J Clin Nutr.* 2008;88(2)558S-564S.

2.Ginde AA, Liu MC, Camargo CA Jr. Demographic differences and trends of vitamin D insufficiency in the US population, 1988-2004. *Arch Intern Med.* 2009;169(6):626- 632.

3. Prentice A. Vitamin D deficiency: a global perspective. *Nutr Rev.* 2008; 66(10 suppl 2): S153-164.

4. Bischoff-Ferrari H et al. Current recommended vitamin D may not be optimal. *Am J Clin Nutr.* 2006; 84:18-28.

5. Vieth R, Bischoff-Ferrari H, Boucher BJ, Dawson- Hughes B, Garland CF, Heaney RP, et al. The urgent need to recommend an intake of vitamin D that is effective. *Am J Clin Nutr* 2007; 85:649-50.

6. Holick MF, Shao Q, Liu WW, et al. The vitamin D content of fortified milk and infant formula. *N Engl J Med.* 992;326(18):1178-81.

7. Jones G. The pharmacokinetics of vitamin D. *Am J Clin Nutr.* In press.

8. Shepard RM, DeLuca HF. Plasma concentrations of vitamin D3 and its metabolites in the rat as influenced by vitamin D3 or 245-hydoxyvitamin D3 intakes. *Arch Biochem Biophys* 1980;202:43-53.

9. Holick MF. Vitamin D deficiency. *N Engl J Med* 2007;357:266-81.

Chapter **13**

Vitamin B12 Supplementation

People with Graves' disease are at risk of Vitamin B12 deficiency due to the following reasons:

In order for Vitamin B12 in food to absorb, we need another substance, called <u>intrinsic factor</u> (IF), which is synthesized by specialized cells in the stomach, called parietal cells. <u>Intrinsic factor</u> (IF) then combines with the ingested Vitamin B12, which is also called the <u>extrinsic factor</u>. The combination of the intrinsic factor and the Vitamin B12 (IF-B12) then travels through the intestines, until it reaches the terminal part of the intestine, which is known as the terminal ileum. Here this <u>IF-B12 </u>complex gets absorbed into circulation.

People with Graves' disease are at increased risk to develop *antibodies* which destroy the parietal cells. This condition is called *atrophic gastritis*. As the parietal cells are destroyed, there is no longer production of Intrinsic factor (IF). In some individuals, antibodies directly attack IF. Lack of IF leads to impaired absorption of Vitamin B12, which manifests as anemia. This is what we call pernicious anemia.

In addition, patients with Graves' disease may also have Ulcerative Colitis or Crohn's Disease, which often involves the terminal ileum, the part of the intestine where Vitamin B12 normally gets absorbed. Consequently, there is further impairment with the absorption of Vitamin B12.

Why Is Vitamin B12 Important?

Vitamin B12 is important for the synthesis and regulation of DNA in every cell of the body. In this way, it is important in maintaining the integrity of our genome.

It is particularly important for the health of the brain, nerves, blood cells, gastrointestinal tract, heart and fatty acids metabolism.

What Are The Symptoms Of Low Vitamin B12?

Low Vitamin B 12 can cause:

1. Lack of energy

2. Tingling and numbness in the feet and hands due to peripheral neuropathy

3. Memory loss

4. Dementia

5. Depression

6. Abnormal gait and lack of balance

7. Anemia

8. Burning of the tongue, poor appetite

9. Constipation alternating with diarrhea, vague abdominal pain

10. Increase in the level of Homocysteine, which is a risk factor for heart disease, stroke, Alzheimer's dementia and bone fractures in the elderly. Low folic acid, Vitamin B6 and genetics are the other contributory factors for raised Homocysteine level.

Who Is At Risk For Low Vitamin B12?

1. Those with gastrointestinal disorders such as atrophic gastritis as I explained above. Also, those with chronic pancreatitis, small intestinal resection or bypass, gluten enteropathy, Crohn's disease and Ulcerative Colitis.

2. Anyone on a strict vegetarian diet, because vegetables are devoid of Vitamin B12.

3. Anyone on the anti-diabetic drug Metformin (Glucophage).

4. Anyone on stomach medicines such as Prilosec, Prevacid, Protonix, Aciphex, Pepcid, Zantac, Tagamet, etc.

5. Antibiotics can lower Vitamin B12 by interfering with the normal intestinal bacterial flora.

6. Anyone who has undergone stomach surgery.

Vitamin B12 Deficiency Often Remains Undiagnosed.

Vitamin B12 deficiency often remains undiagnosed because physicians generally don't think of it as a possibility.

For example, when a diabetic patient complains of tingling in their feet, physicians do all the work-up to diagnose diabetic peripheral neuropathy. They then start you on drug treatment without checking your Vitamin B12 level, even if you are on metformin. In reality, peripheral neuropathy in diabetic patients on metformin is often due to two factors: diabetes itself and Vitamin B12 deficiency.

Vitamin B 12 Deficiency Can Be Diagnosed By A Blood Test.

A blood level less than 400 pg/ml indicates Vitamin B12 deficiency. In my clinical experience, patients do much better when their Vitamin B12 level is close to 1000 pg/ml.

What Are Natural Sources Of Vitamin B12?

Animal products are the main natural sources of Vitamin B12. Plant derived food is *devoid* of Vitamin B12. Good dietary sources include egg yolk, salmon, crabs, oysters, clams, sardines, liver, brain and kidney. Smaller amounts of Vitamin B12 are also found in beef, lamb, chicken, pork, milk and cheese.

Is There Danger Of Vitamin B12 Overdose?

To my knowledge, there are no reported cases of Vitamin B12 overdose in medical literature.

What Are The Different Forms Of Vitamin B12 Supplements?

Vitamin B12 supplements are available as oral pills and pills for sublingual (under the tongue) absorption.

I prefer the sublingual absorption route because the absorption of Vitamin B12 from the oral cavity (dissolving in the mouth) is excellent, better than from the stomach and intestines.

Vitamin B12 is also available in the form of an injection. You need a prescription from a physician for a Vitamin B12 injection.

Chapter **14**

Judicious Use of Anti-Thyroid Drugs

Nature heals slowly. Therefore, I do not leave my patients at risk for the harmful effects of hyperthyroidism, while we are making a U-turn with stress management, dietary changes, Vitamin D and B12 supplementations.

I use anti-thyroid drugs <u>judiciously</u>. Usually, I use Methimazole (Tapazole), because it has a long half life of 4-6 hours. Therefore, it can be taken once or twice a day, as compared to PTU (PropylThioUracil) which has a half life of 75 minutes and therefore, needs to be taken three times a day.

I use PTU in pregnant patients, because Methimazole can potentially cause a serious skin condition in newborns called Cutis aplasia, which is a defect in the skin of a newborn. It is often small and localized to the scalp, but it can be anywhere on the body and can occur as multiple skin defects. I also use PTU in patients who are allergic to Methimazole.

The Starting Dose Of Anti-Thyroid Drugs

I use <u>smaller</u> doses of anti-thyroid drugs, compared to what is generally recommended. These doses work in my patients, because I also take care of the root cause, the autoimmune dysfunction, by changing their mind set, their eating habits and adding Vitamin D and B12 supplements. Perhaps, this is why I have not seen any cases of toxicity due to these drugs in my patients. The starting dose of an anti-thyroid drug depends upon the severity of hyperthyroidism. Here is the usual starting dose of anti-thyroid drugs that I use in my practice.

Initial Dose of Anti-thyroid Drugs

	Mild	Moderate	Severe
Methimazole	5 mg a day	5 mg twice a day	10 mg twice a day
PTU	50 mg twice a day	50 mg three times a day	100 mg three times a day

Outside the US, Carbimazole is used widely. It gets converted to Methimazole in the blood. Roughly 10 mg of Carbimazole yields about 6 mg of Methimazole.

Duration Of Anti-thyroid Drug Treatment

In the traditional practice of Endocrinology, it is recommended to use anti-thyroid drugs no longer than two years. Then, the drug should be stopped. If a person develops recurrence of hyperthyroidism, then the patient should be given an alternative treatment: radioactive iodine or surgery. The two year limit has been arbitrarily chosen for *no* sound reason.

I used to follow this guideline before I developed my own strategy. I realized that if you do *not* treat the underlying auto-immune dysfunction, treatment with an anti-thyroid drug alone is superficial and sub-optimal. I also realized that different individuals respond to treatment differently. Therefore, now I do not follow any rigid guidelines. I treat every patient as a *unique* individual.

My new treatment strategy not only uses anti-thyroid drugs, but also takes care of the root cause of Graves' disease: the autoimmune dysfunction. With this treatment approach, I find some patients need an anti-thyroid drug for a brief period of a few months, while others require it for a longer period. I do not have any *arbitrary* time limit to the use of an anti-thyroid drug.

Side-effects of Anti-Thyroid Drugs

The side-effects of anti-thyroid drugs in discussed in detail in Chapter 7, Traditional Treatment of Graves' Disease.

Chapter 15

Graves' Eye Disease (Orbitopathy, Ophthalmopathy)

Graves' eye disease is medically called Orbitopathy or Ophthalmopathy. Like most endocrinologists, I like the term orbitopathy, because the disease is really behind the eye, but inside the socket of the eyeball or the orbit.

Graves' orbitopathy usually develops concurrently with the onset of hyperthyroidism. However, it can develop months or even years before or after the symptoms of hyperthyroidism.

There are <u>four</u> known factors that can precipitate Graves' orbitopathy:

- Stress
- Cigarette smoking
- Radio-iodine for the treatment of Graves' hyperthyroidism
- Surgery for the treatment of Graves' hyperthyroidism

How Frequent Is Graves' Orbitopathy?

It depends which criteria is used to diagnose Graves' orbitopathy. On ultrasound, CT or MRI scans, changes of Graves' orbitopathy are seen in the vast majority (60-90%) of patients with Graves' hyperthyroidism. However, clinically only about 25-50% of patients with Graves' hyperthyroidism experience Graves' orbitopathy.

Symptoms Of Graves' Orbitopathy

- Retraction of the upper eyelid, giving rise to "stare" look
- Bulging eyes, which is medically termed proptosis or exophthalmos
- Inability to close eyes completely, medically termed lagophthalmos
- Dry, irritated eyes, which give rise to the feeling of a foreign body in the eye. As a reflex, there is excessive tearing.
- Reddened eyes
- Sensitivity to light, medically termed photophobia
- Intense pain in the eye, usually due to corneal ulceration
- Pressure/pain behind the eye
- Double vision
- Decreased vision
- Visual field defects

How Does Graves' Orbitopathy Develop?

Let me first give you a brief overview of the anatomy of the orbit. The orbit is the bony structure or the socket in which the eyeball is located. It is shaped like a pyramid with its base forwards and apex backwards.

Behind the eyeball, there is a space, retro-ocular space, filled with fat, blood vessels, nerves, connective tissues and six muscles of eye movements, known as extra-ocular muscles: They are medial, lateral, superior and inferior rectus muscles and superior and inferior oblique muscles. These muscles are responsible for moving the eye in different directions. There is also another muscle known as levator palpebrae superioris, which elevates the upper eyelid.

Activated Lymphocytes in patients with Graves' disease infiltrate the orbit through the blood vessels. Their target is a cell type called fibroblast, present in the fatty/connective tissue behind the eyeball (retro-ocular fatty/connective tissue) as well in the extra-ocular muscles. Fibroblasts get activated and start to express an otherwise *hidden* antigen, which is recognized by the lymphocytes as *foreign.* This leads to a cascade of events, leading to inflammation and swelling of the soft tissues in the retro-ocular space.

Think of activated lymphocytes as *hyped up* soldiers looking for the enemy, but there is no enemy. Think of fibroblasts as innocent victims, who get scared and start to run after seeing the soldiers. This simply *energizes* the soldiers. They start to cause *damage* and also call for *reinforcement,* as they mistakenly think they have found the enemy.

The fibroblasts then produce an increased amount of matrix, medically known as GlycosAminoGlycan or GAG, which is mainly hyaluronic acid. This matrix *imbibes* water and swells up. The net result is an increased volume of connective tissue behind the eyeball as well as in the extra-ocular muscles.

Activated lymphocytes also produce a number of chemicals, called cytokines, such as interferon gamma, tumor necrosis factor alpha and interleukins. These cytokines cause inflammation and swelling of the soft tissues (connective tissues, fat and extra-ocular muscles) in the retro-ocular space.

The orbit is a bony structure. Therefore, it cannot expand. Thus, the net result of pressure from the increased, swollen, inflamed soft tissues behind the eyeball is to push the eyeball forward, causing the clinical features of <u>bulging </u>of the eyes (proptosis or exophthalmos). Swollen, extra-ocular muscles do not function properly, resulting in <u>double vision</u>. Swollen, retro-ocular soft tissues also compress on the venous return, which contributes to edema (swelling) and congestion of the conjunctiva, which causes reddened eyes.

As eyes are pushed forward, they cannot close completely, which causes the cornea to dry up. That's why eyes feel dry, irritated and sensitive to light. As a reflex, there is excessive tearing. Exposure of the eyes can lead to *abrasions/ulceration* of the cornea (exposure Keratitis), which causes intense eye pain. In severe cases, it can seriously damage the cornea, leading to blindness.

In severe cases of Graves' orbitopathy, crowding of the swollen extra-ocular muscles at the apex of the orbit can compress the optic nerve and damage it. This leads to optic neuropathy. Loss of color vision is the *earliest* sign of optic neuropathy. Other features include decreased eyesight, blind spots in the field of vision or concentric narrowing of the field of vision.

Chronic activation of fibroblasts can eventually lead to fibrosis/scarring of the retro-ocular connective tissue, extra-ocular muscles and levator palpebrae superioris muscle. Scarred, extra-ocular muscles become stiff and can lead to permanent strabismus, resulting is permanent double vision. Scarred, levator palpebrae superioris muscle can lead to permanently retracted upper eyelid, causing cosmetic disfigurement.

Why Does The Immune System Attack The Orbit?

As you may recall, in Graves' disease, activated lymphocytes mount an attack on TSH receptors in the thyroid gland and produce stimulating antibodies, which then command the thyroid cells to produce increased amounts of thyroid hormone.

As it turns out, TSH receptors are also present on the fibroblasts in the retro-ocular fatty/connective tissue and the extra-ocular muscles (1). Activated lymphocytes in patients with Graves' disease *chase* TSH receptors and end up mounting attacks on the fatty-connective tissue present in the orbit of susceptible individuals.

This also explains why Graves' orbitopathy often worsens after patients with Graves' hyperthyroidism are treated with radio-active iodine, which acts by damaging the thyroid cells. Subsequently, TSH receptor protein gets released in circulation, reaches the eyeball and further enhances the attack by the activated lymphocytes. The same mechanism explains worsening of Graves' orbitopathy after thyroid surgery.

Treatment Of Graves' Orbitopathy

Graves' orbitopathy should be treated by an experienced endocrinologist and an experienced ophthalmologist.

Aim of Treatment

1. Relief of symptoms

2. Prevent corneal damage

3. Recognize and treat emergencies such as optic neuropathy, severe proptosis and retro-ocular pain.

4. Corrective and Cosmetic surgery if and when needed.

Most cases of Graves' orbitopathy are mild and improve spontaneously. These patients require simple measures such as artificial tears, glasses to protect eyes from dust and dark glasses if there is light sensitivity. Taping the eyelids closed at night is also helpful.

In moderate to severe cases, oral prednisone is given to reduce the inflammation. It usually requires rather prolonged courses of prednisone, which can cause serious side-effects, such as osteoporosis, increased risk of infections, elevation in blood glucose, etc.

Sometimes radiation is employed with or without prednisone to treat optic neuropathy.

Surgery is needed in some patients. Three types of surgery are carried out in the following order:

1. Decompression surgery. One or more walls of the orbit are removed to relieve intra-orbital pressure. The main indication for decompression surgery is optic neuropathy. Other indications include severe bulging of eyes, retro-ocular pain, peri-orbital pain and intolerable side-effects from prednisone.

2. Strabismus surgery to improve/correct double vision.

3. Eyelid surgery to improve/correct the retracted eyelids and also for cosmetic reasons.

The timing and decision to operate varies from case to case. Graves' orbitopathy usually worsens in the first six months or so. Then, it may improve or become stable. Therefore, it is recommended to wait, unless vision is threatened.

As a general rule of thumb, surgery should be deferred until the patient has achieved a normal thyroid hormone level. The only exception to this rule is severe orbitopathy and threatened vision, in which case decompression surgery is carried out immediately to relieve the intra-orbital pressure.

References:

1. Williams GR. Extrathyroidal expression of TSH receptor. *Ann Endocrinol* (Paris). 2011 Apr;72(2):68-73.

Chapter 16

Graves' Disease and Pregnancy

Graves disease, like other autoimmune diseases, is rare during pregnancy. Why? Because nature is very intelligent. During pregnancy, the immune system becomes very *tolerant*, as it has to *accept* an organism *different* from itself, growing inside the body.

New cases of Graves' disease occur at a rate of about 2 cases per 1000 pregnancies. If you have Graves' disease before pregnancy, it often gets better during pregnancy. However, that is not always the case. Sometimes, patients can develop serious hyperthyroidism and its complications. In addition, their fetus is also at increased risk of complications.

Risks To The Mother

Patients with Graves' disease usually tolerate mild hyperthyroidism pretty well, but moderate to severe hyperthyroidism can cause high blood pressure, eclampsia and congestive heart failure.

Risks To The Fetus

Thyroid hormone from the mother does not cross the placenta. Therefore, even if a mother has a high level of thyroid hormone, it does not affect the fetus. However, Thyroid Antibodies can cross the placenta after about 20 weeks of pregnancy and can affect the fetus.

In Graves' disease, these Thyroid Antibodies are usually stimulating antibodies, known as Thyroid Stimulating Immunoglobulin (TSI). These antibodies can stimulate the fetal thyroid gland (just as they do the maternal thyroid gland) to produce excess thyroid hormone, which results in hyperthyroidism in the fetus as well as in the newborn for the first few months. Fortunately, fetal hyperthyroidism is rare. It occurs in about 5% of mothers with Graves' disease (1).

Rarely, these Thyroid Antibodies may be blocking antibodies (TSH-Stimulation Blocking Antibody or TSBAB) and can lead to hypothyroidism in the fetus as well as in the newborn for the first few months. This occurrence is very rare, affecting only 1 out of 180,000 newborn babies in North America (2).

Hyperthyroidism in the fetus can cause miscarriage, intrauterine growth retardation, prematurity, fetal tachycardia (fetal heart rate > 160 beats per minute) and fetal goiter, which can be detected on an ultrasound.

Hyperthyroidism in the newborn may manifest as irritability, tachycardia, failure to thrive, goiter, bulging eyes, jaundice and low platelet count. It usually occurs a few days after birth if the mother has been receiving anti-thyroid drugs during pregnancy because the maternal anti-thyroid drug crosses the placenta and treats fetal hyperthyroidism. After delivery, it takes a few days for the anti-thyroid drug to disappear in the newborn and then hyperthyroidism manifests itself.

Hyperthyroidism in the newborn resolves spontaneously in a few months, as Thyroid Stimulating Immunoglobulin (TSI) acquired from the mother gradually disappears. However, it may need treatment with anti-thyroid drugs for a short term.

Diagnosis

Diagnosis of Graves' hyperthyroidism during pregnancy is a bit challenging, because many clinical features of pregnancy and hyperthyroidism are similar, such as nervousness, increased sweating, palpitations and shortness of breath. Some features such as goiter, weight loss and Graves' orbitopathy are helpful to diagnose Graves' disease. However, you need laboratory testing to confirm its diagnosis.

These diagnostic blood tests are: Free T4, Free T3, TSH and TSI. In Graves' hyperthyroidism, TSH is below the normal range and is often suppressed. Free T4 and Free T3 are typically elevated, but may be in the normal range in mild cases. TSI is typically elevated.

Gestational Hyperthyroidism

It is important to differentiate hyperthyroidism due to Graves' disease from a *transient* condition during pregnancy, known as Gestational Hyperthyroidism, which is typically due to Hyperemesis Gravidarum. What is Hyperemesis Gravidarum? It is basically a severe form of morning sickness. It usually subsides by the end of the first trimester of pregnancy and with that, Gestational Hyperthyroidism subsides as well. On the other hand, hyperthyroidism due to Graves' disease persists throughout the pregnancy. However, Hyperemesis Gravidarum and its associated Gestational Hyperthyroidism may persist into the second trimester and in some cases, into the third trimester.

Gestational Hyperthyroidism is believed to be due to a hormone from the placenta, called HCG (Human Chorionic Gonadotropin), which can mildly stimulate TSH receptors in the thyroid gland and give rise to hyperthyroidism. HCG is also the culprit for morning sickness.

Rarely, Gestational Hyperthyroidism may be due to molar pregnancy, which is an obstetrical condition in which placental tissue grows into a mass in the uterus. A fetus may or may not be present.

How To Differentiate Between Graves' Disease And Gestational Hyperthyroidism

Goiter, signs of Graves' orbitopathy and an elevated TSI helps to differentiate Graves' disease from Gestational Hyperthyroidism.

Management Of Graves' Disease During Pregnancy

You should be under the care of an endocrinologist if you are diagnosed with hyperthyroidism during pregnancy or if you have a history of Graves' disease or Hashimoto's thyroiditis, even if your blood test for thyroid function is normal. Why? Because even if your hyperthyroidism is under control, your Thyroid antibodies may still be elevated and can cause thyroid issues in your fetus.

Typically, a person with Graves' disease in the U.S. receives Radio-active Iodine, which often controls the hyperthyroidism, but not the autoimmune process. Therefore, these patients often continue to have elevated Thyroid antibodies. Unfortunately, the patient as well as the physician are under the wrong impression that the Graves' disease is cured. When such a patient gets pregnant, often the patient is not referred to an endocrinologist and thyroid antibodies are not even checked. Sad, but true.

If you receive Radio-active Iodine for the treatment of Graves' disease, you should not get pregnant for at least six months in order to prevent radiation-induced risk to your fetus.

During pregnancy, you should ask your physician to refer you to an endocrinologist, who should check and monitor your Thyroid Antibodies, especially during the second half of the pregnancy, when these antibodies can cross the placenta and cause thyroid issues in the fetus.

Specific Treatment Of Graves' Disease

While you need to discuss the specific treatment of your Graves' disease and hyperthyroidism with your physician, here are some general guidelines, which most endocrinologists agree upon.

1. Radio-active Iodine treatment must **Never** be carried out during pregnancy.

2. Anti-Thyroid drugs are the main specific treatment of Graves' disease during pregnancy.

3. Thyroid surgery is considered only rarely if there is a serious concern of toxicity from anti-thyroid drugs. In that case, partial thyroid removal, known as subtotal thyroidectomy, is carried out. The surgery should be scheduled in the second trimester to avoid the increased risk of miscarriage from anesthesia in the first trimester and the risk of premature labor in the third trimester.

4. How much Anti-thyroid drug should be given? The aim of the anti-thyroid drug should be to bring Free T4 and Free T3 into the upper limit of the normal range. Over-treatment with anti-thyroid drugs can increase the risk of <u>fetal hypothyroidism</u>, because anti-thyroid drugs cross the placenta and can decrease fetal thyroid hormone production.

5. It is important to closely monitor the patient with Free T4, Free T3 and TSH on a 1-2 months basis. Thyroid antibodies, TSI (Thyroid Stimulating Immunoglobulin) or TRAB (Thyrotropin Receptor Antibody) should be tested at about <u>24</u> weeks of pregnancy and monitored on a case by case basis.

6. Pregnancy in a Graves' disease patient should be regarded as high risk and a perinatologist should be involved if thyroid antibodies are found to be elevated.

Are Anti-Thyroid Drugs Safe During Pregnancy?

Every drug can have potential side-effects. For this reason, the general rule of thumb is **Not** to use any drug during pregnancy if possible. However, if hyperthyroidism is left untreated, it can be harmful to the mother as well as the fetus.

Anti-thyroid drugs used in North America are PTU (Propylthiouracil) and MMI (Methimazole, also available with the brand name, Tapazole).

In Europe and some other regions of the world, Carbimazole is widely used. Carbimazole converts into Methimazole in the body.

Side-Effects Of Anti-thyroid Drugs

<u>To the Mother</u>

Anti-thyroid drugs are old drugs. Propylthiouracil and Methimazole were approved in 1947 and 1950, respectively (1).

They are generally well tolerated, but rarely, side-effects may develop. These side-effects can be *minor* such as itching, skin rash, joint pains and stomach upset. *Major side effects include* liver toxicity, vasculitis (inflammation of blood vessels) and granulocytopenia (a decrease in the number of white blood cells). Granulocytopenia is usually transient, but in some cases, it can progress to suppression of bone marrow, termed agranulocytosis, which is a serious medical condition and can be fatal.

Liver toxicity and vasculitis are more common with PTU (Propylthiouracil) than with Methimazole. Liver toxicity occurs rarely, in about 0.1 % of cases. In 2009, the FDA (the Food and Drug Administration) issued an alert regarding PTU-induced Liver injury. Its Adverse Event Reporting System (AERS) has identified 32 cases of serious liver injury associated with the use of PTU over the past 20 years. Among them, 22 were adults and 10 were children. Among these adults, 12 deaths and 5 liver transplants took place. Among children, 1 death and 6 liver transplants occurred. In contrast, 5 cases of serious liver injury were identified with the use of methimazole. All five cases were in adult patients and 3 resulted in death (1). PTU treatment during pregnancy resulted in two cases of serious maternal liver injury and there were two cases of liver injury in fetuses whose mothers took PTU (2). The average daily dose of PTU associated with liver failure was approximately 300 mg in both children and adults. Liver failure occurred after 6 to 450 d (median, 120 d) of treatment (2). It is estimated that each year one or two individuals with Graves' disease in the United States will die or require a liver transplant after PTU treatment (2). The risk of PTU-related severe liver failure appears to be higher in children than in adults (2). In conclusion, PTU should be used only if a person cannot take Methimazole. This is particularly true in the case of children.

Symptoms of liver failure include fatigue, weakness, vague abdominal pain, loss of appetite, itching, easy bruising or yellowing of the eyes or skin. If you develop these symptoms, it is best to stop the anti-thyroid drug, inform your physician and have your liver function tested immediately.

Agranulocytosis occurs very rarely, in about 0.02% of cases, which translates into 2 patients out of 10,000. If the drug is stopped, full recovery may or may not take place. It usually develops early in the course of treatment, within 2 months, but can develop even later.

Granulocytopenia and agranulocytosis predisposes an individual to serious life-threatening infections, and can be fatal. Therefore, these drugs should be prescribed only by endocrinologists who are experienced in using these drugs. If you develop fever or severe sore throat, it is best to stop the drug, consult your physician and have your blood tested for <u>white cell count</u>.

If you suspect your anti-thyroid drug is causing any side-effect, immediately contact your physician. It is best to stop the drug and have an appropriate blood test, such as <u>white cell count</u> and <u>liver function test</u>. If these tests are normal, you may want to go back on the anti-thyroid drug, after consulting your physician.

Side-Effects Of Anti-thyroid Drugs

To the Fetus

1. Fetal Hypothyroidism

Anti-thyroid drugs cross the placenta and therefore can affect the thyroid gland of the fetus. There can be a 36% decrease in Free T4 in the newborns of mothers with Graves' disease, whose Free T4 is brought down into the <u>lower two-thirds</u> of the normal range during pregnancy with anti-thyroid drugs (3). Therefore, it is a common endocrine practice to *prevent* overtreatment of hyperthyroidism during pregnancy. Most endocrinologists simply bring Free T4 into the upper normal range.

2. Birth defects

Methimazole can pose a potential risk of three birth defects: Cutis aplasia, choanal atresia and esophageal atresia. <u>Cutis aplasia</u> is a defect in the skin, usually affecting the scalp. <u>Choanal atresia</u> implies a blockage in the back of the nasal passages. <u>Esophageal atresia</u> is a defect in the distal part of the esophagus, which ends in a blind-ended pouch, instead of connecting to the stomach.

Therefore, In general, endocrinologists use PTU to treat Grave's disease during pregnancy, especially during the *first* trimester when organ formation (organogenesis) is taking place and consequently, the risk of birth defects is high. After the first trimester, the FDA recommends to switch from PTU to Methimazole

(1), in view of a relatively high risk of liver failure with PTU as compared to Methimazole.

What About Beta-Blockers?

Beta-blocker drugs such as propranolol or atenolol are commonly used in hyperthyroid patients to slow down heart rate and tremors. During pregnancy, beta-blockers should be used cautiously and only for a short period. In addition to potential risk to the mother, such as exacerbation of asthma, bradycardia (slow heart rate) and low blood pressure, beta-blockers can cross the placenta and lead to fetal bradycardia (slow heart rate), decreased response to anoxia (lack of oxygen) and a low blood glucose in the newborn.

What Should I Do?

Obviously, there is a lot to consider before you decide to go on a particular anti-thyroid drug. Educate yourself on this important subject and find an experienced endocrinologist who can customize an individual treatment plan tailored to your needs and preferences.

My Treatment Strategy To Treat Graves' Disease During Pregnancy

I treat Graves' disease in pregnant patients pretty much the same way as I treat Graves' disease in non-pregnant patients, with special emphasis on the points already elaborated in this chapter. As already discussed in detail, my treatment strategy consists of:

- Stress management without medications.
- Special Diet for Graves' disease.
- Vitamin D supplementation.
- Vitamin B12 supplementation.
- Judicious use of anti-thyroid drugs.

Please refer to Chapter 9 for a detailed description of my strategy to treat Graves' disease.

Let me emphasize two points:

1. Stress Management is even more important during pregnancy. The news of having Graves' disease can be unnerving, because now you have to worry about your baby as well.

2. Vitamin D supplementation becomes even more important. Why? Because your fetus cannot synthesis its own Vitamin D and is entirely dependent on you for its supply. Therefore, I closely monitor the 25 OH Vitamin D level in my patients with Graves' disease during their pregnancy, following the same principles I discussed earlier in the book.

See Chapter 12, "Vitamin D Supplementation" for more information. For a detailed, in depth discussion regarding Vitamin D, please refer to my book, "Power of Vitamin D."

References:

1.http://www.fda.gov/Drugs/DrugSafety/PostmarketDrugSafetyInformationforPatientsandProviders/DrugSafetyInformationforHeathcareProfessionals/ucm162701.htm

2. http://jcem.endojournals.org/content/94/6/1881.full#ref-7

3. Azizi F, Amouzegar A. Management of hyperthyroidism during pregnancy and lactation. Eur J Endocrinol. 2011 Jun;164(6):871-6.

Chapter **17**

Case Studies

Case Study 1

A 35 year old Caucasian female initially saw her gynecologist for symptoms of excessive sweating, heat intolerance, insomnia, emotional swings, decreased libido, tremors and palpitations.

She thought she might be going through menopause. Her gynecologist ran a bunch of blood tests, including thyroid function test, which turned out to be abnormal.

Her gynecologist appropriately advised her to see an endocrinologist. That's why she decided to consult me.

I found that she had a small goiter and mild, bilateral exophthalmos. I ordered blood tests for thyroid function which turned out as follows:

	Patients' Lab. Result	Normal Range
TSH	< 0.05	0.4 - 4.50 mIU/L
Free T4	2.23	0.8 - 1.8 ng/dL
Free T3	6.84	2.3 - 4.2 pg/ml
Thyroglobulin Antibody	250	< 20 IU/ml
Thyroid Peroxidase Antibody	4091	<35 IU/ml

As you can see, her TSH was suppressed, Free T4 as well as Free T3 levels were elevated. These tests confirmed that she had hyperthyroidism. Now let's look at her Thyroid antibody levels. Both were elevated, which confirms that the reason for her hyperthyroidism was her autoimmune dysfunction. Therefore, I diagnosed her with hyperthyroidism due to Graves' disease.

I counseled her about the treatment options for Graves' disease. She opted for my treatment strategy. She was going through a very stressful time in her life. In addition, she was experiencing a lot of stress from the political scene. It was back in 2004. She was a Democrat and an anti-Iraq war activist.

I did extensive stress management. I also placed her on my diet, Vitamin D supplement and Tapazole (methimazole) 5 mg three times a day. Within a few days, she developed generalized skin itching without any rash. I switched her from Tapazole to PTU 50 mg three times a day, which she tolerated well and did not have any side-effects. One month later, she was feeling better.

Two months later, her Free T4 and Free T3 were normal, but TSH was still very low. Six months later, her TSH also normalized. Please note that TSH lags behind the normalization of Free T3 and Free T4. Once TSH is suppressed, it takes several months of normal Free T3 and Free T4 before TSH rises back into the normal range.

Once her TSH had normalized, I decreased her PTU to 50 mg twice a day. Fifteen months later, I decreased her PTU to 50 mg once a day. Twenty six months later, I stopped her PTU altogether.

I also found her blood level of Vitamin B12 to be in the low normal range. I placed her on Vitamin B12 lozenges for sublingual absorption.

Through this twenty six months period, I continued to monitor her liver function and white cell count on a 2-3 months basis and these tests remained normal. She continued to feel good. All of her symptoms had vanished and her exophthalmos did not worsen.

I continued to monitor her closely with thyroid function test every 2 - 3 months. Twelve months after stopping PTU, her TSH went low as 0.03 mIU/L, Free T3 went slightly high as 478 pg/ml, although Free T4 was normal as 1.6 ng/dL. I diagnosed her with recurrence of hyperthyroidism due to Graves' disease and placed her on PTU 50 mg twice a day.

Please note that in hyperthyroidism due to Graves' disease, initially it is only Free T3 that gets elevated; Free T4 rises later. TSH gets down due to a rise in Free T3 and/or Free T4.

Two months later, her Free T3 was normal, but TSH was still low. Five months later, her TSH normalized. Twelve months later, I stopped her PTU and increased Vitamin D to 2000 IU per day from 1000 IU per day.

Three months after stopping PTU, her TSH was normal as 1.66 mIU/L. But at four months, it went low as 0.03, although her Free T3 and Free T4 were in the normal range. Her 25 OH Vitamin D level was 65 ng/ml (normal range 30-100 ng/ml). She told me that she had recently started a new job and had been under a lot of stress. I decided **not** to restart her on PTU. Instead, I did extensive stress management, increased Vitamin D to 4000 IU a day from 2000 IU a day.

I saw her again in two months and by that time, her TSH became normal as 1.65 mIU/L. Since then, I have increased her dose of Vitamin D to 6000 IU a day and she reads my book, "Stress Cure Now" on a regular basis.

It has been over four years since stopping her PTU. She continues to do well. Her Free T4, Free T3 and TSH continue to be normal and Vitamin D level stays in the upper normal range, on a dose of 6000 IU per day.

Lessons To Learn:

- Symptoms of hyperthyroidism may mimic Menopause.
- Stress precipitates hyperthyroidism.
- If skin reaction develops due to Tapazole, switch to PTU.

- Once TSH is suppressed, it takes several months of normal Free T3 and Free T4 before TSH rises back into the normal range.
- My treatment strategy not only controls hyperthyroidism effectively, but it also prevents any progression of Graves' eye disease.

Case Study 2

A 58 year old Caucasian female was referred to me by her Gastroenterologist, as she was found to have a very low TSH during her work-up for chronic diarrhea of 2 years duration. Patient also had symptoms of heat intolerance, weight loss and excessive urination.

On my examination, I found that she had a small goiter. I ordered a blood test for thyroid function, the results of which showed that her TSH was suppressed, but her Free T3 and Free T4 were in the normal range.

Sometimes a person may have low TSH level, but normal Free T3 and Free T4 levels. In traditional endocrinology, we call it subclinical hyperthyroidism, which in my opinion is a misleading term, as it implies that you have hyperthyroidism, but no clinical symptoms due to it. In fact, most of these individuals have clinical symptoms of hyperthyroidism. Therefore, I like to say that these individuals are suffering from mild hyperthyroidism, instead of subclinical hyperthyroidism.

I diagnosed her with mild hyperthyroidism due to Graves' disease and placed her on my treatment strategy. I put her on Tapazole 5 mg a day in addition to my diet, Vitamin D supplement and stress management.

Two months later, her diarrhea had resolved, her TSH was normal and remained normal for the rest of her clinical course. Nine months later, I decreased her Tapazole to 2.5 mg a day. Sixteen months later, I decreased it further to 2.5 mg every other day. At

<u>twenty one months</u>, I stopped her Tapazole, but continued to monitor her thyroid function.

More than <u>five years</u> later, she continues to have normal thyroid function, without any anti-thyroid drugs.

Lesson To Learn:

I selected this case study to point out how hyperthyroidism can masquerade as a gastrointestinal disease. Many physicians with a myopic approach stay focused on a gastrointestinal diagnostic work-up, but don't find an answer. The patient may suffer for years before a physician with a more comprehensive approach orders a blood test for TSH.

Case Study 3

A 53 year old Caucasian female, was referred to me by her Primary Care Physician for abnormal thyroid function, which were as follows:

	Patients' Lab. Result	Normal Range
TSH	< 0.01	0.4 - 4.50 mIU/L
Free T4	6.1	0.8 - 1.8 ng/dL
Free T3	18.51	2.3 - 4.2 pg/ml
Thyroglobulin Antibody	< 20	< 20 IU/ml
Thyroid Peroxidase Antibody	15	<35 IU/ml

Her TSH was suppressed, Free T4 and free T3 markedly elevated, but her Thyroglobulin Antibodies and Thyroid Peroxidase

Antibodies were NOT elevated. She started having symptoms of fatigue, hyperhidrosis, palpitations, shakiness and weight loss for about 2-3 months.

She had been having a lot of anxiety since the death of her father about 4 months ago and was on an anti-anxiety drug. On my clinical examination, she had a small goiter, mild bilateral exophthalmos and a fine tremor in her hands. She had clinical features of hyperthyroidism and her Thyroid Function Test confirmed it. However, did she have Graves' disease in the absence of an elevation of Thyroglobulin Antibodies and Thyroid Peroxidase Antibodies? I thought so.

In order to confirm my clinical impression, I ordered Radioiodine uptake and scan of thyroid, which showed that her Radioiodine uptake by the thyroid gland was *markedly* elevated as 70% at 6 hours and 88% at 24 hours. In addition, the uptake was diffuse, without any hot or cold nodules. These findings confirmed my clinical impression that she had hyperthyroidism due to Graves' disease.

I started her on Tapazole 5 mg three times a day. I also added Atenolol 25 mg three times a day to control her palpitations and tremors. Her 25 OH Vitamin D level was very low at 12 ng/ml. So I started her on Vitamin D 5000 IU twice a day. I also did extensive stress management.

One month later, she was feeling great. All of her symptoms of hyperthyroidism had resolved. Her Free T3 and Free T4 had come down into the normal range and her TSH was still suppressed. I decreased the dose of Tapazole to 5 mg twice a day and Atenolol to 25 mg twice a day.

Nine months later, I decreased her Tapazole to 5 mg in the morning and 2.5 mg in the evening. Thirteen months later, I decreased her Tapazole to 5 mg a day.

Twenty four months later, she had mild elevation in Free T3 and Free T4, as she was under a lot of stress. I increased her Tapazole to 5 mg in the morning and 2.5 mg in the evening. Twenty five months later, her Free T3 and Free T4 were back to normal and she was feeling great.

Twenty Nine months later, which is the at the time of this writing, she continues to do well and is on Tapazole 5 mg a day.

Lessons To Learn

- Anti-anxiety drugs may help to control your symptoms of anxiety, but do not take care of the underlying root cause of anxiety: fear. Therefore, it is very superficial approach and does not prevent autoimmune disorder.

- Some patients with Graves' disease do not have elevated Thyroglobulin Antibodies and Thyroid Peroxidase Antibodies. In these cases, the next step is to do a Radioiodine uptake and scan of thyroid or one can do a blood test for Thyroid Stimulating Immunoglobulin (TSI).

- Response to treatment varies from patient to patient. Some need an anti-thyroid drug for a shorter duration, while others need it for a longer duration. Why? Because each one of us is so unique in our genetics, biochemistry, eating habits and psychosocial makeup.

Case Study 4

A 59 year old Caucasian male started having palpitations, agitation, tremors, nervousness, frequent bowel movements and weight loss over a six month period. He was under severe stress due to his professional responsibilities. Then, he developed double vision when he looked downwards, for which he consulted an ophthalmologist and a neurologist at the teaching hospital of a prestigious medical school. He underwent extensive testing, including a MRI of his brain, echocardiogram of his heart and doppler test of his neck arteries, all of which turned out to be normal. Apparently, a thyroid function test was **not** done. His double vision resolved spontaneously.

Later, he started to see an internist, who did get his TSH which was low as 0.01. Apparently, the patient was **not** told that he had hyperthyroidism.

Eighteen months later, his TSH was even lower as <0.01, but apparently he was **not** told that he had hyperthyroidism. Another fifteen months went by and he continued to suffer from palpitations, agitation, tremors, nervousness, and frequent bowel movements.

Finally, he had another blood test done which showed that his TSH was suppressed. Free T3, Free T4, Thyroglobulin Antibodies and Thyroid Peroxidase Antibodies were all elevated.

At this juncture, he saw an endocrinologist, who ordered a Thyroid Radioiodine uptake and scan, which showed that his 6 -hour uptake was elevated at 31.9% and 24 hour uptake was elevated at 42%.

His endocrinologist recommended radioactive iodine ablation for his Graves' disease. However, he was not convinced that was the right strategy. With the help of his wife and the internet, he found me.

When I sew him, he was still having palpitations, agitation, nervousness, fine tremors, heat intolerance and frequent bowel movements. He told me that he used to have asthma during his childhood. On my examination, I found a goiter in his neck.

I put him on my strategy to treat Graves' disease. For an anti-thyroid drug, I chose Tapazole 10 mg twice a day. He was already on a beta-blocker, Toprol 100 mg a day, which I continued.

Two months later, all of the symptoms that had haunted him for three years resolved. His Free T3 and Free T4 came down into the normal range.

Six months later, his TSH had also normalized. At this point, I lowered his Tapazole to 10 mg in the morning and 5 mg in the evening. Eight months later, his TSH was elevated as 19.9, but his Free T3 and Free T4 were normal and he was feeling fine. I further lowered his Tapazole to 2.5 mg twice a day.

Ten months later, his TSH, Free T3 and Free T4 were all normal. Fifteen months later, his TSH was getting elevated as 4.2, so I decreased his Tapazole to 2.5 mg a day and continued it for another twenty four months, during which time he continued to have normal TSH, Free T3 and Free T4. After a total of thirty nine months since the initiation of treatment, I stopped his Tapazole.

His Thyroid function remained normal over the next 6 years. Then, his TSH became slightly elevated as 6.98 and he was also feeling tired. His Free T4 and Free T3 were normal. His internist told him the usual presumptive explanation physicians have been taught: Oh! your thyroid gland is now "burnt out," which means you will have to be on thyroid hormone for the rest of your life.

I ordered a full panel of thyroid antibodies to figure out whether his hypothyroidism was due to a destructive process in the thyroid gland called Hashimoto's thyroiditis or due to antibodies interfering with the action of TSH.

His Thyroglobulin Antibodies and Thyroid Peroxidase Antibodies were normal, indicating he did not have Hashimoto's thyroiditis. His TBII (Thyrotropin Binding Inhibit Immunoglobulin) was slightly elevated as 22% (normal is < 16) and his TSI (Thyroid Stimulating Immunoglobulin) was negative, which meant that his hypothyroidism was due to antibodies that block TSH from acting on its receptors on the thyroid cells. It was good news with a good long term prognosis. Very likely his hypothyroidism will be mild and transient.

It is interesting to note that this patient refused to increase his Vitamin D intake to more than 4000 IU a day. His 25 OH Vitamin D level has stayed in the range of 40-60 ng/ml, although I would like to see it in the 80-100 ng/ml range. He also continues to pursue his high stress career and has not fully embraced my approach to deal with stress.

Lessons To Learn:

- The diagnosis of hyperthyroidism and Graves' disease may be missed even in the best hands.

- Graves' orbitopathy causing double vision may be transient and the diagnosis will be missed if a thyroid function test is not ordered.

- Always ask for a TSH blood test if the cause of your symptoms is not readily apparent.

- Always ask for copies of your blood test. Ask your physician to explain if TSH is abnormal. If you are not satisfied with the explanation, see an endocrinologist.

- You can develop hypothyroidism even when your Graves' disease has been in remission for years.

- Ask your physician to properly evaluate the cause of your hypothyroidism, instead of just presuming that it is a "burnt out" thyroid. You should ask for the following blood tests: Thyroglobulin Antibodies, Thyroid Peroxidase Antibodies, TBII (Thyrotropin Binding Inhibit Immunoglobulin) and TSI (Thyroid Stimulating Immunoglobulin).

- Elevated Thyroglobulin Antibodies and Thyroid Peroxidase Antibodies indicate that you have a destructive process, Hashimoto's thyroiditis, going on in your thyroid gland and you are at risk of gradually losing all of your thyroid gland, the so called burnt out thyroid, if you don't take the proactive approach discussed in this book to calm your immune system down.

- Elevated TBII (Thyrotropin Binding Inhibit Immunoglobulin) and negative TSI (Thyroid Stimulating Immunoglobulin) means that your Graves' disease is in remission, but you have developed antibodies which are *blocking* the action of TSH on the thyroid cells. You can get rid of these antibodies and cure your hypothyroidism by adhering to my treatment strategy to treat immune dysfunction, discussed in this book.

- Elevated TBII (Thyrotropin Binding Inhibit Immunoglobulin) and positive TSI (Thyrotropin Stimulating Immunoglobulin) means that your Graves' disease is still active.

Case Study 5

A 67 year old Caucasian female started having excessive weight loss without any change in her eating habits. She got concerned and saw her primary care physician, who did a blood test for thyroid function, which was consistent with the diagnosis of Hyperthyroidism.

The patient was referred to an endocrinologist, who diagnosed her with Graves' disease. Somehow, her primary care physician also ordered a thyroid Ultrasound which showed a 1.4 centimeter nodule in the right lobe. The physician then ordered a thyroid radioiodine uptake and scan, which showed that her 6-hour as well as 24-hour uptakes were markedly elevated, again confirming that she had Grave's disease, although the overzealous radiologist interpreted it as a "toxic multinodular goiter" and recommended radioiodine therapy. Her nodule was again noticed on the Scan as a functioning nodule.

It is interesting to note that a month prior, her endocrinologist had already established through the blood work-up that she had Graves' disease. However, somehow the primary care physician decided to do thyroid ultrasound as well as a thyroid uptake and scan, neither of which added anything more to the diagnosis. If anything, the radiologist's diagnosis of a "toxic multinodular goiter" was incorrect.

Her endocrinologist placed her on Tapazole 10 mg twice a day. Three weeks later, she developed severe Migraine headaches, for which she took an anti-Migraine medicine, Imitrex, which did not help much. In the past, Imitrex had helped her Migraine headaches effectively. So the patient stopped Tapazole on her own and her Migraine headache subsided. Then, she restarted Tapazole at 10 mg a day, but soon her Migraine headache recurred with great intensity and lasted one week. She stopped Tapazole and her Migraine headache abated. She got dissatisfied with her endocrinologist and primary care physician, switched to another primary care physician and decided to seek a second endocrine consultation. That's how she came to see me. At that time, she was off Tapazole for four weeks.

She was having symptoms of fatigue, excessive perspiration and shakiness. She was very nervous, confused and apprehensive. Her Thyroid function test results were as follows.

	Patients' Lab. Result	Normal Range
TSH	< 0.01	0.4 - 4.50 mIU/L
Free T4	2.7	0.8 - 1.8 ng/dL
Free T3	8.26	2.3 - 4.2 pg/ml
Thyroglobulin Antibody	2,266	< 20 IU/ml
TSI (Thyroid Stimulating Immunoglobulin	219	<125 % baseline

Her 25 OH Vitamin D level was 34 ng/ml, while taking vitamin D3 as 2000 IU per day.

She had been under a lot of stress due to a number of physical and psychological reasons. She had a long history of Migraine headaches which were under control with Imitrex. She also suffered from chronic insomnia and took sleeping pills. Four years prior, she was diagnosed with stomach cancer and had part of her stomach removed. She suffered from severe low back pain for many years and took pain medications. She also took multiple supplements per her naturopath. She was diagnosed with osteoporosis three years ago. In addition, she was a life-long activist for certain political and social issues, which added tremendously to her own stress.

I discussed my treatment strategy with her. I did extensive stress management, increased her Vitamin D to 4000 IU per day, discussed my Low Carbohydrate Diet and started her on PTU 100 mg three times a day. She was reluctant to take PTU, as she had read all of the bad publicity on the internet about the side-effects of PTU. She also did not want Radioiodine therapy or surgery. On my reassurance, she decided to give PTU a try.

At two weeks, she developed an episode of Migraine headache, but it was less severe than the one with Tapazole and it responded well to Imitrex. She got scared and stopped PTU. I told her to restart PTU at a smaller dose of 50 mg three times a day, which she tolerated well, without any recurrence of Migraine headaches.

She had also started having pain in the eyes and double vision. She saw an ophthalmologist, who diagnosed her with Graves' orbitopathy and started her on oral Prednisone 40 mg a day, tapering it by 10 mg every week. When I saw her, she was having bilateral exophthalmos (right worse than the left), inflammation of conjunctiva and watery eyes. I concurred with the diagnosis and treatment of Graves' orbitopathy.

At six weeks, her Free T4 and Free T3 came down into the high normal range and her TSH was still less than 0.02. Her Prednisone was down to 10 mg a day and her eye pain, which initially improved, had recurred. I increased her Prednisone back to 20 mg a day and tapered it more slowly, by 5 mg every 2 weeks. I also increased her dose of Vitamin D3 to 6000 IU per day.

On each visit, I also did extensive stress management. She read my book, "Stress Cure Now" and started to understand the basis of stress and how one can be free of it, without medications.

At eight weeks, her Free T3 and FreeT4 had further come down and her TSH was now 0.12. I decreased her PTU to 50 mg twice a day. Her eye pain and inflammation had improved. I increased Vitamin D3 to 8000 IU per day and continued on tapering doses of Prednisone.

Over the next several weeks, her eye pain and inflammation continued to improve. Then, she saw a Graves' orbitopathy specialist at a prestigious teaching hospital, who concurred with the treatment.

At four months, her TSH was 0.64, with Free T4 and FreeT3 in the low normal range. I further decreased her PTU to 50 mg a day and increased her Vitamin D3 to 10,000 IU per day. By now, she was on Prednisone 5 mg a day, which I further reduced to 2.5 mg a day, alternating with 5 mg a day for 2 weeks, then down to 2.5 mg a day.

At five months, she was feeling much better, except for the watery eyes. She was gaining weight. Her TSH was 1.3, Free T3 and Free T4 were in the low normal range and she was on PTU 50 mg a day. Her 25 OH Vitamin D level was 69 ng/ml on Vitamin D3 at a dose of 10,000 IU per day. I further increased her Vitamin D3 to 12,000 IU per day and decreased her Prednisone to 2.5 mg a day.

At seven months, I ordered a repeat thyroid ultrasound, which again showed a 1.4 cm nodule in the Right lobe of the thyroid. I then ordered an Ultrasound guided Fine Needle Aspiration Biopsy of this nodule, which turned out to be benign. Interestingly, her Thyroid function test done two weeks after the biopsy had worsened: her TSH went down to less than 0.01, Free T3 increased to 4.9 and Free T4 went up, but still in the normal range. Perhaps, the stress in the form of worrying about the biopsy and the physical trauma from the biopsy itself triggered worsening of her autoimmune dysfunction. I did extensive stress management and increased her dose of PTU to 50 mg three times a day. Within a month, her Free T3 came down into the normal range.

At nine months, she had come off Prednisone completely. Therefore, I decreased the dose of Vitamin D3 to 8000 IU per day. She was feeling well except for the pronounced bulging (exophthalmos) and excessive watering of the right eye and the double vision. I cleared her for Decompression surgery of the right eye, which was carried out successfully by her Graves' disease ophthalmologist.

At fourteen months, her watery eye and double vision had improved. I continued her at PTU 50 mg three times a day for the next fourteen months, during which time her Free T3, Free T4 and TSH remained normal.

At twenty five months, she had intermittent double vision, only in bright florescent light and while watching TV or a stage show. She saw her ophthalmologist, who performed right eye lid cosmetic surgery to improve her pronounced right eye exophthalmos, with good cosmetic results.

At twenty eight months, I tested her for TSI (thyroid stimulating Immunoglobulin) which turned out to be negative, which meant that her Graves' disease was in remission. Therefore, I stopped her PTU. Four months later, at the time of this writing, she continues to do well, with normal TSH, Free T3 and Free T4.

During this period of treatment, her Vitamin D intake varied between 6000 IU to 12,000 IU per day, mostly at 8000 IU per day and she weighs about 115-120 Lbs. On this dose of Vitamin D, her 25 OH Vitamin D level remained in the range of 60-90 ng/ml. Remember, she had most of her stomach removed after she was diagnosed with stomach cancer. People with stomach surgery require larger doses of vitamin D supplement.

I also kept her on Vitamin B12 sublingual lozenges, 1000 microgram three times a day for two reasons: She had stomach surgery and she had Graves' disease. Both of these conditions are associated with low vitamin B12.

Lessons To Learn

- Stress, especially in the form of worrying, is a precipitating factor for Graves' disease.

- Once you are diagnosed with Graves' disease, make sure you are under the care of an endocrinologist. Let him/her decide which tests to order.

- Some Primary Care Physicians, especially in the US, may order unnecessary tests for fear of litigation. This "shooting in the dark" approach is not only unnecessary, costly and potentially harmful, but also may put you on the wrong track.

- Some over-zealous radiologists may interpret more than what they see. Radiologists do not see the patients, but the screen. Therefore, be careful when a radiologist gives a clinical diagnosis, which may be incorrect. This case study is a good example, because the radiologist diagnosed her with a Toxic Multinodular Goiter and recommended radioactive iodine therapy. If she did not come to see me, her primary care physician might have sent her for radioactive iodine therapy for the treatment of "Toxic Multinodular Goiter." Not only she would have been misdiagnosed, but radioactive iodine treatment could have resulted in a severe case of Graves' orbitopathy that was already in the making.

- Graves' orbitopathy can start after a patient has been hyperthyroid for some time. It usually worsens in the first few months, as happened in this case. During this time, oral Prednisone can be helpful for ameliorating the inflammation of the eyes. While on Prednisone (or any other steroid), patients should also receive high doses of Vitamin D supplement to counteract the negative effects of Prednisone, especially on the bones.

- Patients with Graves' disease and orbitopathy should preferably be treated by endocrinologists and ophthalmologists who have expertise in treating Graves' disease.

- Patients with stomach surgery and those on steroids, such as Prednisone, require larger doses of Vitamin D supplements to keep their blood level of 25-OH Vitamin D in the optimal range of 50-100 ng/ml.

- TSI (thyroid stimulating Immunoglobulin) blood test can be used to assess the clinical progress of Graves' disease patients. When TSI becomes negative, it indicates that Graves' disease is in remission. Anti-thyroid drugs can be stopped at that point.

PART TWO

RECIPES

Recipes

This section contains a number of my original recipes. Sounds shocking! A doctor talking about recipes. I understand your shock.

Let me share my own journey regarding cooking. Until the age of about 35, I did not know much about cooking. My cooking skills were limited to making a cup of tea, an omelet and toast. Then, my mother came to live with me, as she had become disabled due to a stroke. Back then, there was no Indian restaurant in my town. As a necessity, I started cooking at home, because she did not care for regular American food. As I would cook, my mother would also be in the kitchen in her wheelchair, giving instructions, step by step. The results were pretty good. It encouraged me and I started to like cooking.

As an endocrinologist, I realized the important role food plays in our health. I clearly see we are what we eat. Gradually, I got more and more involved in cooking. I did *not* follow any cook books. I simply followed the basic principles of Indian cooking I learned from my mother and improvised my own recipes.

Now, I love cooking. With the help of my lovely wife, we even grow our own vegetables, herbs and fruits. We also have our own chickens. They are great pets because they lay eggs, keep the yard fertilized, eat snails and children love them. You don't have to have a rooster for hens to lay eggs, a fact many people don't know.

It is such a pleasure to just walk into the back yard and pick fresh vegetables and herbs. While cooking breakfast, I bath in the morning sun, while doing yoga and meditation at the same time. Actually, cooking keeps you in the Now and whenever you are in the Now, you are meditating. The purpose of meditation is to shift your attention into the Now.

Each and every one of these recipes has been subjected to the taste buds of my wife and some friends. I hope you enjoy them too.

Bon appetite!

BREAKFAST SUGGESTIONS

Yogurt

Put 3-4 tablespoons of Plain, Regular yogurt in a bowl. Add a handful of blueberries, blackberries, raspberries or raisins and walnuts, pecans, shredded almonds or pine nuts. Mix well. You can also add 1-2 tablespoons of honey if you like it sweet.

Feta Cheese

Take 2-3 tablespoons of feta cheese. Add black olives and pine nuts, walnuts or pecans. Optional: You can add mint leaves or basil leaves.

Hard Boiled Eggs

Peel and slice two hard boiled eggs and one Avocado. You can sprinkle salt, black pepper or cayenne pepper, according to your taste.

Tip: You can prepare a few "hard-boiled eggs" ahead and keep them in the refrigerator for a handy, quick snack.

Caution: Use hard-boiled eggs within a few days, definitely within a week or they will spoil.

Omelets

Basic Omelet

Cooking Time = About 10 minutes

Ingredients:

Eggs = 2 (egg whites only)
Green onions = 2 (You can use 1/2 of one regular white onion in place of green onions), chopped
Olive oil = 2 tablespoons
Salt = ½ teaspoon

Add olive oil and chopped onions to a medium or large pan. Place it on stove at low heat. Cook for a few minutes until onions have softened and turned yellowish.

Meanwhile, crack open 3 eggs in a bowl. Using a tablespoon, dish out 1 egg yolk and throw it away. Leave one egg yolk. Beat it along with the egg whites. Add the eggs to the pan once onions are done.

Sprinkle the salt. In a few minutes, the eggs start looking like an omelet. With a spatula, turn the omelet over. Don't worry if it breaks down. Just turn the pieces over. Cook for a few minutes and your delicious Omelet is ready.

Mushroom Omelet

Follow the basic omelet recipe, but use a handful of mushrooms after your onions are done. Follow the rest of the recipe.

Spinach Omelet

Follow the basic omelet recipe. Add a handful of washed spinach leaves soon after you pour the beaten eggs in the pan. Cook another couple of minutes. Then fold it, instead of turning it over, so the spinach is all inside. Let it cool off for 2-3 minutes, before you eat.

Bell Pepper Omelet

Follow the basic omelet recipe. Chop 1/2 of a bell pepper (any color) and add when you start with your onions. If you like spicy, you can add ½ teaspoon of Cumin seeds and ¼ to ½ teaspoon of cayenne pepper or black pepper soon after pouring the eggs.

Add a few fresh leaves of cilantro or parsley. Then fold it over, so the chopped bell pepper is all inside. Let it cool off for 2-3 minutes, before you eat.

Avocado Omelet

Peel an avocado and slice it into chunks. Once the basic omelet is ready, add avocado chunks. Add a few fresh leaves of cilantro or parsley. Then fold it over, so the avocado chunks are all inside. Let it cool off for 2-3 minutes, before you eat.
If you like avocados, this will be a morning delight for you. Avocados help to raise your good (HDL) cholesterol and are a good source of protein.

Spicy Omelet

Follow the basic omelet recipe. Right after you add the eggs to the pan, add ¼ to ½ teaspoon of cayenne pepper. Add ½ teaspoon of Cumin seeds. Add a few fresh leaves of cilantro or parsley. You can also use ½ of a jalapeño pepper in place of cayenne pepper.

Scrambled Eggs - Mushrooms

Cooking Time = About 10 minutes

Ingredients:

Eggs = 1-2 (egg whites only)
Mushrooms = 4, diced
Green onions = 2 or a small regular onion, chopped
Garlic = 1 clove, chopped
Olive oil = 2 tablespoons
Salt = 1/2 teaspoon

Optional:

Fenugreek seeds = 1/2 teaspoon
Cumin seeds = 1/2 teaspoon
Turmeric = 1/2 teaspoon
Clove = 1/4 teaspoon
Cayenne pepper = 1/2 teaspoon OR ½ of a jalapeño, sliced
Mustard, yellow or Dijon = 1/2 teaspoon

In a pan, add olive oil, onions, garlic and salt. Start the stove at low heat and let it cook for about 5 minutes, stirring frequently. Then, add mushrooms and let it cook for another few minutes.

In a bowl, crack open 1 - 2 eggs, beat well and add to the pan. Let cook for a few minutes, stirring frequently. Cool for a couple of minutes before serving.

Optional:

In the beginning, add turmeric, fenugreek seeds, cumin seeds and clove along with the onions. At the end, you can add few cherry tomatoes, fresh cilantro or parsley leaves, fresh mint leaves or fresh basil leaves.

Make it Spicy: In the beginning, add ¼ to ½ teaspoon of cayenne pepper or ½ of a jalapeño pepper in place of cayenne pepper.

Scrambled Eggs - Spinach

Cooking Time = About 10 minutes

Ingredients:

Eggs = 1-2 (egg whites only)
Spinach = about 1/2 cup
Green onions = 2 or a small regular onion, chopped
Garlic = 1 clove, chopped
Olive oil = 2 tablespoons
Salt = 1/2 teaspoon

Optional:

Cranberries, fresh or dried = a handful
Fenugreek seeds = 1/2 teaspoon
Cumin seeds = 1/2 teaspoon
Turmeric = 1/2 teaspoon
Clove = 1/4 teaspoon
Cayenne pepper = 1/2 teaspoon or ½ of a jalapeño pepper in place of cayenne pepper
Mustard, yellow or Dijon = 1/2 teaspoon

In a pan, add olive oil, onions, garlic and salt. Start the stove at low heat and let it cook for about 5 minutes, stirring frequently. Then add spinach and let it cook for another few minutes.

In a bowl, crack open 1 - 2 eggs, beat well and add to the pan. Let cook for a few minutes, stirring frequently. Cool for a couple of minutes before serving.

Optional:

In the beginning, add a few cranberries, turmeric, fenugreek seeds, cumin seeds and clove, along with onions. At the end, you can add cherry tomatoes, fresh cilantro or parsley leaves, fresh mint leaves or fresh basil leaves.

Make it Spicy: In the beginning, add ¼ to ½ teaspoon of cayenne pepper OR ½ of a jalapeño pepper.

Scrambled Eggs - Spinach - Eggplant - Bell Pepper

Cooking Time = About 15 minutes

Ingredients:

Egg = 1-2 (egg whites only)
Spinach = about 1 cup
Eggplant = 1, preferably Japanese or Chinese, chopped
Bell pepper = 1, any color, preferably red, cut into chunks
Tomatoes = 5 cherry, halved or 1 regular, cut into chunks
Green onions = 2 or a small regular onion, chopped
Garlic = 1 clove, chopped
Mustard, yellow or Dijon = 1 tablespoon
Apple cider vinegar = 1 teaspoon
Olive oil = 2 tablespoons
Salt = 1/2 teaspoon

Optional:

Pine nuts = a handful
Fenugreek seeds = 1/2 teaspoon
Cumin seeds = 1/2 teaspoon
Turmeric = 1/2 teaspoon
Cayenne pepper = 1/2 teaspoon OR ½ of a jalapeño pepper

In a pan, add olive oil, onions, garlic and salt. Start the stove at low heat and add eggplant. Pour mustard and vinegar on eggplant chunks. Cook for about 5 minutes, stirring frequently.

In a bowl, crack open 1 - 2 eggs, beat well and add to the pan. Let cook on low heat for a few minutes, stirring frequently. Once eggs are done, add spinach, tomatoes and bell pepper. Cook for 3-5 minutes on low heat.

<u>Optional:</u>
In the beginning, add turmeric, fenugreek seeds and cumin seeds along with onions. In the end, add pine nuts, fresh cilantro or parsley leaves, fresh mint leaves or fresh basil leaves.

Make it Spicy: In the beginning, add ¼ to ½ teaspoon of cayenne pepper OR ½ of a jalapeño pepper along with onions.

Scrambled Eggs - Bell Pepper - Zucchini

Cooking Time = About 15 minutes

Ingredients:

Eggs = 1-2 (egg whites)
Bell pepper = 1/2 diced
Zucchini = 1/2 small, chopped
Tomato = 1, diced
Green onions = 2 or a small regular onion, chopped
Garlic = 1 clove, chopped
Olive oil = 2 tablespoons
Salt = 1/2 teaspoon

Optional:

Fig = 1, ripe
Fenugreek seeds = 1/2 teaspoon
Cumin seeds = 1/2 teaspoon
Turmeric = 1/2 teaspoon
Clove = 1/4 teaspoon
Cayenne pepper = 1/2 teaspoon OR ½ of a jalapeño, sliced
Mustard, yellow or Dijon = 1/2 teaspoon

In a pan add olive oil, zucchini, onions, garlic and salt. Start the stove at low heat and let it cook for about 5 minutes, stirring frequently. Then, add bell pepper and cook for another few minutes.

In a bowl, crack open 1 - 2 eggs, beat well and then add to the pan. Let cook for a few minutes, stirring frequently. Cool for a couple of minutes before serving.

Optional:

In the beginning, add turmeric, fenugreek seeds, cumin seeds, and clove, along with onions. At the end you can add few cherry tomatoes, fresh cilantro or parsley leaves, fresh mint leaves.

Make it Spicy: In the beginning, add ¼ to ½ teaspoon of cayenne pepper OR ½ of a jalapeño pepper and add about 1/2 teaspoon of yellow mustard.

Make it Sweet: At the end, add one ripe fig and fresh basil leaves.

Scrambled Eggs - Bell Pepper - Cauliflower

Cooking Time = About 20 minutes

Ingredients:

Eggs = 1-2, (egg whites only)
Bell pepper = 1/2 of regular sized bell pepper, any color. Cut into several pieces
Cauliflower = 1/8 of the whole cauliflower head, chopped into 4-6 small pieces
Onion = 1/2 of a medium sized onion, chopped
Garlic = 1 clove, sliced
Olive oil = 3 tablespoons
Vinegar = 1/2 teaspoon
Lemon, fresh = Cut in half
Dijon Mustard (or regular, yellow) = small amount
Salt = 1/2 teaspoon

Optional:

Pine nuts = a handful
Cumin seeds (or powder) or Caraway seeds = 1/2 teaspoon
Turmeric powder = 1/2 teaspoon
Clove powder = 1/4 teaspoon
Black pepper OR Cayenne pepper = 1/2 teaspoon
Cilantro or Basil or Mint leaves = 8 -10

In a regular frying pan, pour 1 cup of water. Add mustard and salt. Squeeze the juice of 1/2 lemon. Stir. Place it on the stove at medium heat. Add cauliflower and cover it. Let it cook for about 10 minutes. Check only once or twice to make sure the water has not cooked off. Avoid frequent uncovering. It will reduce the amount of steam, which is cooking the cauliflower.

Uncover, lower the heat. Add olive oil, onion, and garlic.

Stir frequently. DO NOT COVER. In about 3-5 minutes, when there is very little water left, add one or two beaten eggs. Scramble it with the spatula. Let it cook for about 3-5 minutes, until eggs are done. Stir frequently.

Add bell pepper and cook for another 3-5 minutes. In the end, add vinegar, a handful of pine nuts and cilantro, basil or mint leaves. Mix well.

Optional: In the beginning, add clove powder, turmeric powder, cumin (or caraway seeds), black pepper OR cayenne pepper.

Scrambled Eggs - Bell Pepper - Green Beans

Cooking Time = About 15 minutes

Ingredients:

Eggs = 1-2 (egg whites only)
Bell pepper = 1 diced
Green Beans = 10
Tomato = 1, diced
Green onions = 2 or a small, regular onion, chopped
Garlic = 1 clove, chopped
Olive oil = 2 tablespoons
White Vinegar = 1/2 teaspoon

Optional:

Cranberries, fresh or dried = a handful
Fenugreek seeds = 1/2 teaspoon
Cumin seeds = 1/2 teaspoon
Turmeric = 1/2 teaspoon
Cayenne pepper = 1/2 teaspoon OR ½ of a jalapeño

In a pan, add a small amount of water and olive oil. Add green beans, onions and garlic. Start the stove at medium heat and let cook for about 5 minutes, stirring frequently. Do not cover. Then, add tomatoes, bell pepper and white vinegar. Let cook for another few minutes.

In a bowl, crack open 1 - 2 eggs, beat well and add to the pan. Let cook for a few minutes, stirring frequently. Cool for a couple of minutes before serving.

Optional:
In the beginning, add cranberries, turmeric, fenugreek seeds and cumin seeds along with onions. At the end, you can add fresh oregano or thyme leaves.

Make it Spicy: In the beginning, add ¼ to ½ teaspoon of cayenne pepper OR ½ of a jalapeño pepper.

Scrambled Eggs - Green Beans - Eggplant

Cooking Time = About 20 minutes

Ingredients:

Eggs = 1-2, (egg whites only).
Green beans = 15
Eggplant = 1/2, preferably Japanese or Chinese.
Cinnamon stick = 1
Tomato = 1, medium size
Yogurt = Plain, 2-3 tablespoons
Garlic = 1 clove, sliced
Olive oil = 3 tablespoons
Lemon, fresh = Cut into two halves
Dijon Mustard (or regular, yellow) = small amount
Salt = 1/2 teaspoon

Optional:

Pine nuts = a handful
Bay leaf = 1
Cumin seeds (or powder) or Caraway seeds = 1/2 teaspoon
Turmeric powder = 1/2 teaspoon
Cloves powder = 1/4 teaspoon
Black pepper OR Cayenne pepper = 1/2 teaspoon
Cilantro or Basil or Mint leaves = 8-10

In a regular frying pan, pour 1/2 cup of water. Add mustard and salt. Squeeze 1/2 lemon. Stir and cook at <u>medium</u> heat. Add green beans, eggplant, cinnamon stick and bay leaf. DO NOT COVER. Let cook for about <u>5</u> minutes. Stir occasionally. Lower the heat. Add olive oil, garlic, yogurt and tomato.

Stir frequently. DO NOT COVER. In about <u>10</u> minutes, add one or two beaten eggs. Scramble it with a spatula. Let it cook for another 3 - 5 minutes, until eggs are done. Stir frequently. In the end, add a handful of pine nuts and cilantro leaves (or basil or mint leaves).

<u>Optional</u>:

In the beginning, add bay leaf, clove powder, turmeric powder, cumin (or caraway seeds), powdered black pepper (or powdered cayenne pepper).

Scrambled Eggs - Bell Pepper - Zucchini - Daikon Radish

Cooking Time = About 15 minutes

Ingredients:

Eggs = 1-2 (egg whites only)
Bell pepper = 1/2, diced
Zucchini = 1/2, sliced
Daikon Radish = 4 inch piece, peeled and cut in small pieces
Green onions = 2 or a small regular onion, chopped
Garlic = 1 clove, chopped
Olive oil = 2 tablespoons
Salt = 1/2 teaspoon

Optional:

Pine nuts = a handful
Fenugreek seeds = 1/2 teaspoon
Cumin seeds = 1/2 teaspoon
Turmeric = 1/2 teaspoon
Clove = 1/4 teaspoon
Cayenne pepper = 1/2 teaspoon OR ½ of a jalapeño, sliced
Mustard, yellow or Dijon = 1/2 teaspoon
Cherry tomatoes = 5-8
Fresh cilantro, mint or basil leaves = 8-10
Figs = 2 ripe

In a frying pan, add olive oil, zucchini, Daikon radish and onions. Place the pan on stove at low heat.

Optional: Add garlic, turmeric, fenugreek seeds, cumin seeds, and clove.

Sprinkle salt. Let cook for about 5 minutes, stirring frequently. Then, add bell pepper and let cook for another few minutes.

In a bowl, beat 1 - 2 eggs and then add to the pan. Let it cook for a few minutes, stirring frequently. Let it cool for a couple of minutes before serving.

Optional:

At the end, add a few cherry tomatoes, pine nuts, fresh cilantro, mint or basil leaves.

Make it Spicy: In the beginning, add cayenne pepper OR jalapeño pepper and add mustard.

Make it Sweet: Add two ripe figs, chopped and a few fresh basil leaves.

Scrambled Eggs - Pumpkin

Cooking Time = About 15 minutes

Ingredients:

Eggs = 1 - 2 (egg whites only)
Pumpkin, fresh = 10 small slices, about 1/4 inch thick, 2 inches wide and 2 inches long, peeled.
Celery Stick = 1, cut into small pieces
Olive oil = 2 tablespoons
Vinegar = 1/2 teaspoon
Lemon, fresh = Cut in half
Mustard, regular, yellow = small amount
Salt = 1 teaspoon
Cumin seeds (or powder) or Caraway seeds = 1 teaspoon
Garlic = 1 clove, sliced

Optional:

Black Pepper OR Cayenne pepper = 1/2 teaspoon.

A wok works better, but you can use a regular frying pan. Add olive oil, pumpkin and celery slices to the wok. Place it on the stove at medium heat. Stir frequently. DO NOT COVER. In about 10 minutes, pumpkin slices will be done: softened but not mushy.

Turn the heat down to low. Add the mustard and squeeze the juice of 1/2 lemon directly on the pumpkin slices. Add vinegar, garlic, cumin seeds, and salt. Let it cook another 2-3 minutes, stirring frequently.

Add beaten eggs to the wok. After a minute, scramble it. Cook for another 2 - 3 minutes.

Optional:

Make it Hot: In the beginning, add Cayenne OR Black Pepper on the pumpkin slices.

Scrambled Eggs - Green Beans - Bell Pepper - Tomatoes - Turnip

Cooking Time = About 15 minutes

Ingredients:

Eggs = 1-2 (egg whites only)
Green beans = 4-6
Bell pepper = 1/2, diced
Tomatoes = 1-2, diced
Turnip = 1/2, peeled and diced
Green onions = 2 or a small regular onion, chopped
Garlic = 1 clove, chopped
Olive oil = 2 tablespoons
Salt = 1/2 teaspoon
Lemon = Cut in half.

Optional:

Fenugreek seeds = 1/2 teaspoon
Cumin seeds = 1/2 teaspoon
Turmeric = 1/2 teaspoon
Cayenne pepper = 1/2 teaspoon OR ½ of a jalapeño, sliced
Mustard, yellow or Dijon = 1/2 teaspoon
Fresh cilantro leaves = 8-10

In a frying pan, add olive oil, 1/2 cup of water, turnip, onion, garlic, and salt. Squeeze lemon directly onto the pan.

Optional: Add fenugreek seeds, cumin seeds, turmeric, cayenne pepper and mustard.

Cover and cook on low heat for about 10 minutes, stirring occasionally to make sure water is still there. Then, add bell pepper, green beans, and tomatoes. Let it cook for another few minutes, uncovered. Add beaten eggs to the pan. After a minute, scramble it Cook for another 2 - 3 minutes. In the end, add cilantro leaves.

LUNCH OR DINNER

You can use any of the scrambled eggs recipes for lunch or dinner.

Lettuce Wraps: Cheese - Avocado - Eggs - Mango

Ingredients:

Lettuce = 1 head of Iceberg lettuce
Cheese, feta or cottage = a small amount
Avocado = 1, peeled, sliced
Eggs= 2, boiled, peeled, sliced (egg whites only)
Mango (preferably <u>Kent</u> variety from Mexico, available at Indian grocery stores during summer) = 1 ripe, peeled, cut into slices
Salt = a tiny amount

Gently peel off a leaf from the lettuce head. Place the mango slices, cheese, avocado slices and egg slices in the center of the lettuce leaf. Sprinkle a tiny amount of salt. Roll up the lettuce leaf into a wrap. You can make about 4 wraps with this recipe.

SALADS

Salad 1 (Cucumber - Tomato - Yogurt Salad)

Ingredients:

Yogurt, plain = 4 tablespoons
Tomatoes, cherry = 6 - 10
Cucumber = 1 medium sized, cut into pieces
Green Onion = 1 sliced. Also use green portion
Salt = 1/2 teaspoon
Cumin seeds = 1/2 teaspoon
Mint leaves or basil leaves (preferably fresh) = a few

     Add yogurt to a medium sized bowl. Dilute it by adding and mixing 2 tablespoons of water. Then, add onion, cucumber, cumin seeds, salt and mix well. Then mix in tomatoes and mint leaves. Your salad is ready.

Salad 2 (Cucumber - Tomato - Avocado Salad)

Ingredients:
Lettuce = a few leaves, chopped
Cucumber = 1/2, sliced
Tomato = 1 medium, cut into large pieces OR about 10 cherry tomatoes, whole
Avocado = 1, peeled, sliced
Onion = regular, 1/2, peeled, cut into slices
Mint leaves or Cilantro leaves = a few, preferably fresh
Balsamic Vinegar = a tiny amount
Lime or Lemon = 1, cut in half
Salt = a tiny amount

     In a medium size bowl, add chopped lettuce. Then, add chopped onion, tomatoes and avocado. Mix well. Add mint or cilantro leaves. Sprinkle salt and a tiny amount of Balsamic Vinegar. In the end, squeeze lime. Mix well.

Salad 3 (Olive - Pine Nut - Avocado Salad)

Ingredients:

Olives, black or green = 8-10
Pine nuts = a handful
Avocado = 1, peeled, sliced
Lettuce = a few leaves, chopped
Tomato = 1 medium, cut into large pieces OR about 10 cherry tomatoes, whole
Balsamic Vinegar = a tiny amount
Lime or Lemon = 1, cut in half
Salt = a tiny amount.

      In a bowl, add chopped lettuce. Squeeze lemon juice and sprinkle salt and a tiny amount of Balsamic Vinegar. Then add pine nuts, olives, tomatoes and avocado. Mix well.

Salad 4 (Papaya - Spinach - Pine Nut Salad)

Ingredients:

Lettuce, Romaine = half cup, chopped
Arugula = half cup, chopped
Spinach, baby = half cup
Cucumber = 1/2, sliced
Papaya = 1, small, peeled, seeds removed and cut into chunks
Tomato = 1, medium, cut into large pieces OR about 10 cherry tomatoes, whole
Pine nuts = a handful
Balsamic Vinegar = a tiny amount
Lime or Lemon = 1, cut in half

      In a bowl, add baby spinach, chopped lettuce and arugula. Squeeze lemon juice and add a tiny amount of Balsamic Vinegar. Then add cucumber, pine nuts and tomatoes. In the end, add papaya. Mix gently.

Pumpkin Z-Fries

Cooking Time = About 15 minutes

Ingredients:

Pumpkin, fresh = Cut into the size of French Fries, about 20 - 25, some peeled and some unpeeled
Olive oil = 2 tablespoons
Cheddar cheese, shredded = a handful
Mustard, Dijon = 3 teaspoons
Vinegar = 1/2 teaspoon

Optional:

Garlic powder = 1 teaspoon
Salt = 1/2 teaspoon
Cumin seeds (or powder) or Caraway seeds = 1 teaspoon
Black Pepper = 1 teaspoon OR Cayenne pepper = 1/2 teaspoon

Place a frying pan on medium heat. Warm olive oil and then, add pumpkin fries. Add Dijon mustard directly on the pumpkin fries.

Optional: Add vinegar, garlic, cumin seeds, salt and black OR cayenne pepper.

Cook for about 10 minutes. DO NOT COVER. Turn the pumpkin fries over a few times, so they don't get burned.

Turn the heat down to low. Sprinkle a handful of shredded cheddar cheese. It will melt in a couple of minutes. Place Pumpkin Z-Fries on paper towel to soak up excess oil.

Pumpkin Z-Fries - Scrambled Eggs - Eggplant

Cooking Time = About 15 minutes

Ingredients:

Eggs = 2 (egg whites only)
Pumpkin, fresh = Cut into the size of French Fries, about 20 - 25, some peeled and some unpeeled
Eggplant = 1 Japanese or Chinese or 2 small round ones; sliced
Olive oil = 3 tablespoons
Cheddar cheese, shredded = a handful
Mustard, Dijon = 3 teaspoons
Vinegar = 1/2 teaspoon

Optional:
Garlic powder = 1 teaspoon
Salt = 1/2 teaspoon
Cumin seeds (or powder) or Caraway seeds = 1 teaspoon
Onion, Green = 2, chopped. (You can use a small regular onion instead)
Black Pepper = 1 teaspoon OR Cayenne pepper = 1/2 teaspoon
Fresh or dried thyme, oregano, mint OR basil leaves

In a pan, add olive oil, pumpkin fries, and eggplant slices. Add mustard directly on the pumpkin fries.

Optional: Add vinegar, garlic, cumin seeds, salt and black or cayenne pepper.

Cook for about 10 minutes on <u>medium</u> heat. DO NOT COVER. Turn the pumpkin fries and eggplant slices over a few times, so they don't get burned. Then, turn the heat down to low. Sprinkle in a handful of shredded cheddar cheese. In a few minutes, add onions and beaten eggs to the pan. Let it cook about 1 minute, then scramble the eggs with a spatula. Cook for another 2 - 3 minutes, stirring frequently. In the end, add fresh or dried oregano, thyme, mint or basil leaves.

Zucchini Z-Fries - Avocado

Cooking Time = About 15 minutes

Ingredients:

Zucchini, fresh = Unpeeled, cut into the size of French Fries, about 20-25
Avocado = 1, peeled, sliced
Cherry tomatoes = about 10
Olive oil = 3 tablespoons
Cheddar cheese, shredded = a handful
Mustard, Dijon = 4-5 teaspoons
Garlic powder = 1 teaspoon
Onion, Green = 2, chopped (You can use a small regular onion instead.)

Optional:

Salt = 1/2 teaspoon
Clove powder = 1/2 teaspoon
Cumin seeds (or powder) or Caraway seeds = 1 teaspoon
Black Pepper = 1 teaspoon OR Cayenne pepper = 1/2 teaspoon
Cilantro leaves = 8-10 fresh or dried = 1 teaspoon

In a regular frying pan, add olive oil and zucchini fries .
Sprinkle garlic powder and add mustard directly on the zucchini fries.

Optional : Add clove powder, cumin seeds, salt and black or cayenne pepper directly on the zucchini fries.

Cook for about 5 minutes on medium heat. DO NOT COVER. Turn the zucchini fries over a few times, so they don't get burned. Sprinkle a handful of shredded cheddar cheese directly on the zucchini fries. Once the cheese melts, remove the zucchini fries onto a plate. Top it with chopped onions, cherry tomatoes, avocado slices and cilantro leaves.

Pumpkin Stir Fry

Cooking Time = About 15 minutes

Ingredients:

Pumpkin, fresh = 10 small slices, about 1/4 inch thick, 2 inches
wide and 2 inches long, peeled
Celery Stick = 1, cut into small pieces
Olive oil = 2 tablespoons
Vinegar = 1/2 teaspoon
Lemon, fresh = Cut in half.
Mustard, regular, yellow = small amount
Salt = 1 teaspoon
Cumin seeds (or powder) or Caraway seeds = 1 teaspoon
Garlic = 1 clove, sliced
Black Pepper = 1 teaspoon OR Cayenne pepper = 1/2 teaspoon

Optional:
Avocado slices
Mint or Basil leaves = 8-10

        A wok works better, but you can use a regular frying pan.
Warm olive oil on medium heat. Add pumpkin slices and celery
slices. Stir frequently. DO NOT COVER. In about 10 minutes, pumpkin
slices will be done: softened but not mushy.

        Turn the heat down to low. Add mustard and 1/2 lemon juice
directly on the pumpkin slices. Add vinegar, garlic, cumin seeds, salt
and cayenne pepper (or black pepper) to the wok. Let it cook another
2-3 minutes, stirring frequently.

Optional:
For variety, add Avocado slices at the end. Let it cook another 2-3
minutes, stirring frequently. In the end, add a few Mint or Basil
leaves.

Cauliflower - Pumpkin - Turnip Stir Fry

Cooking Time = About 15 minutes

Ingredients:

Pumpkin, fresh = 15 small slices, about 1/4 inch thick, 2 inches wide and 2 inches long, peeled
Cauliflower = 3 - 5 florets
Turnip = 1/2, peeled and cut into small slices
Celery Stick = 1, cut into small slices
Olive oil = 2 tablespoons
Vinegar = 1/2 teaspoon
Lemon, fresh = Cut in half
Mustard, regular, yellow = small amount
Salt = 1 teaspoon
Cumin seeds (or powder) or Caraway seeds = 1 teaspoon
Garlic = 1 clove, sliced
Mint leaves Or Basil leaves, fresh = 8-10 OR dried = 1 teaspoon

Optional
Black Pepper = 1 teaspoon OR Cayenne pepper = 1/2 teaspoon

A wok works better, but you can use a regular frying pan instead. Place the wok on <u>medium</u> heat. Add olive oil, pumpkin slices, turnip slices, cauliflower florets and celery slices to the wok. Stir frequently. DO NOT COVER. In about 10 minutes, pumpkin slices will be done: softened but not mushy.

Turn the heat down to low. Add mustard and 1/2 lemon juice directly on the pumpkin slices. Add vinegar, garlic, cumin seeds and salt.

Optional: Add cayenne pepper OR black pepper to the wok.

Let it cook another 2-3 minutes, stirring frequently.

Zucchini - Eggplant - Avocado Delight

Cooking Time = About 15 minutes

Ingredients:

Zucchini = 1 medium size, unpeeled, sliced
Eggplant = 1 small, preferably Japanese or Chinese, sliced
Avocado = 1, peeled, sliced into chunks
Yogurt = Plain, 2 tablespoons
Tomato = 1 medium size, sliced
Onion = 1/2 of a medium sized onion
Olive oil = 3 tablespoons

Optional:

Walnuts or pecans = a handful
Clove, powder = a pinch
Garlic = 1 clove, sliced
Cumin seeds (or powder) or Caraway seeds = 1/2 teaspoon
Turmeric powder = 1/2 teaspoon
Black pepper OR Cayenne pepper = 1/2 teaspoon
Oregano, thyme or rosemary leaves = about 1 teaspoon

In a regular frying pan on medium heat, add olive oil and chopped onions. Stir frequently. In about 3-5 minutes, onion will turn yellowish.

Lower the heat. Add sliced Zucchini and eggplant. After about 2-3 minutes, add yogurt. Let it cook for about 10 minutes on low heat. DO NOT COVER. Stir frequently.

Add Avocado slices and tomato slices. Cook for another couple of minutes. In the end, add walnuts and oregano or thyme or rosemary leaves.

Optional: In the beginning, add clove powder, turmeric powder, cumin (or caraway seeds), black pepper, cayenne pepper.

Eggplant - Bell Pepper - Daikon Radish

Cooking Time = About 15 minutes

Ingredients:

Eggplant = 1 small, preferably Japanese or Chinese, sliced
Bell pepper = 1/2, cut into pieces
Daikon radish = about a 4 inch piece, peeled and cut into pieces
Yogurt = Plain, 2 tablespoons
Tomato = 1 medium size, sliced
Olive oil = 3 tablespoons
Mustard - yellow or Dijon = a small amount

Optional:

Cumin seeds (or powder) or Caraway seeds = 1/2 teaspoon
Turmeric powder = 1/2 teaspoon
Black pepper OR Cayenne pepper = 1/2 teaspoon
Basil or thyme leaves = 8-10

In a regular frying pan, add 1/2 cup of water, olive oil, eggplant and Daikon radish. Put on low heat, cover and stir only a couple of times. In about 5 minutes, uncover and add yogurt and tomato.

Optional: Add cumin (or caraway seeds), black pepper OR cayenne pepper.

Cook for about 5 minutes on low heat. DO NOT COVER. Stir frequently.

Add bell pepper and cook for about 2-3 minutes. Add a small amount of mustard and cook for another 2-3 minutes. In the end, add basil leaves or thyme leaves.

Zucchini - Bell Pepper - Green Beans - Mushroom

Cooking Time = About 15 minutes

Ingredients:

Zucchini = 1, small, unpeeled, sliced
Bell pepper, red = 1, cut into pieces
Green beans = small, 8-10
Mushrooms = white, 5, cut into halves
Tomato = 1 medium, sliced
Onion = 1 small, chopped
Olive oil = 1 tablespoon
Mustard - yellow or Dijon = a small amount
Vinegar, Balsamic = a small amount

Optional:

Cumin seeds (or powder) or Caraway seeds = 1/2 teaspoon.
Turmeric powder = 1/2 teaspoon.
Black pepper OR Cayenne pepper = 1/2 teaspoon.
Basil or Oregano leaves = 8-10

In a regular frying pan, add 1/2 cup of water, olive oil, onion and mustard. Put on low heat, cover and stir only a couple of times. In about 5 minutes, uncover and add green beans, zucchini and tomatoes. _Cook for about 5 minutes on <u>medium</u> heat. DO NOT COVER. Stir frequently.

Then, add bell pepper and mushrooms. Cook for about 2-3 minutes. In the end, add basil leaves or thyme leave and sprinkle with a small amount of vinegar.

Optional:
In the beginning, add cumin (or caraway seeds), black pepper OR cayenne pepper.

Cauliflower, Bell Pepper, Green Beans, Cherry Tomatoes and Green Grapes

Cooking Time = About 15 minutes

Ingredients:

Cauliflower = 1/8 of the whole cauliflower head, chopped into 4-6 small pieces
Bell pepper = 1/2 of regular sized bell pepper, any color. Cut into 4-5 chunks
Eggplant = 1/2 of a Chinese or Japanese eggplant, cut into chunks
Green grapes = about 20
Green Beans, small = 5-10
Cherry Tomatoes = 5-10
Onion = 1/2 of a regular sized onion
Garlic = 1 clove, sliced
Olive oil = 3 tablespoons
Mustard, Dijon, (or regular, yellow) = small amount
Salt = 1/2 teaspoon
Pine nuts = a handful
Cilantro or basil = 1/2 teaspoon

Optional:
Cumin seeds (or powder) or Caraway seeds = 1/2 teaspoon
Turmeric powder = 1/2 teaspoon
Black pepper OR Cayenne pepper = 1/2 teaspoon.

In a regular frying pan on low heat, add olive oil and 1/2 cup of water. Add mustard, salt, cauliflower and eggplant, and cover. Let it cook for about 10 minutes. Check only once or twice to make sure water is still in there. Uncover and raise the heat to medium. Add onion, garlic, cherry tomatoes, green beans and grapes. Stir frequently. DO NOT COVER. Add a handful of pine nuts, and basil OR cilantro leaves.

Optional: In the beginning, add cumin (or caraway seeds), turmeric, black pepper OR cayenne pepper.

5 - Leaf Saag

Cooking time = about 60 minutes

Ingredients:

Spinach, baby = 4 cups, chopped
Mustard greens = 6 cups, chopped
Daikon Radish Leaves = 3 cups, chopped
Arugula = 1 cup, chopped
Turnip Leaves = 1 cup, chopped
Daikon Radish = 1, peeled, chopped
Olive oil = 10 tablespoons
Butter = 1 stick
Onion = 2 medium, chopped
Garlic = 2 cloves, sliced
Vinegar = Any type, preferably Balsamic, 1 teaspoon
Salt = 1 teaspoon
Turmeric powder = 1/2 teaspoon
Cilantro leaves = a few
Lime or lemon = 1, cut in half

Optional:

Cumin seeds = 1 teaspoon
Clove powder = 1/2 teaspoon
Black pepper= 2 teaspoons OR Cayenne pepper = 1 teaspoon

In a large pot, add olive oil. Then add two chopped onions, garlic and salt. Cook on low heat for about 5 minutes, stirring frequently, until the onions have turned yellowish brown.

Add spinach, mustard greens, Daikon radish and Daikon radish leaves, turnip leaves, arugula, turmeric powder, salt and vinegar.

Cook for about 45 minutes at low heat, uncovered, stirring frequently until it is not runny and has thick consistency.

Then, pour it into a blender and grind on low until all leaves are well ground. Pour it back into the large pot.

Add 1 stick of butter. Cook for another 15 - 20 minutes on low heat, uncovered, until you start to see oil separating at the periphery.

In the end, add cilantro. Squeeze and add lime or lemon. Mix well. Let it sit for about 15 minutes before serving.

<u>Optional</u>:
In the beginning, add black pepper OR cayenne pepper and clove powder and cumin seeds.

MEAT DISHES

Chicken Nuggets
(Kids and teenagers love them)

Cooking Time = About 30 - 45 minutes

Ingredients:

Chicken = Boneless, preferably breast, about 1 Lb., cut into pieces about 2 x 1 inches
Yogurt = 3 tablespoons
Olive oil = 2 tablespoon
Lime or lemon = 1, cut in half
Apple cider vinegar = 1 teaspoon
Mustard, Dijon = 1 teaspoon
Garlic powder = 1 tablespoon
Sea-Salt = 1 teaspoon

Optional:

Cayenne pepper or black pepper = 1/2 teaspoon

In a large pan, add olive oil, yogurt, apple cider vinegar, Dijon mustard, garlic powder and salt. Squeeze lime or lemon into it. Add 3 tablespoons of water. Mix well.

Optional: Sprinkle Cayenne pepper or black pepper and mix well.

Marinate chicken nuggets in the pan for about 15 - 30 minutes.

Place the pan on medium heat. Stir frequently. Cook nuggets on medium heat for about 5 - 10 minutes, until all yogurt is dried out. Lower the heat and cook for another 5 minutes, until nuggets have turned golden in parts.

Chicken - Bell Pepper

Cooking Time = About 15 minutes

Ingredients:

Chicken = 2 chicken breasts, cut into chunks or 4 drumsticks
Bell pepper = 2 medium, any color, preferably red, cut into chunks
Olive oil = 4 tablespoons
Celery: 1 stick, sliced into small pieces
Onion = 2 medium, chopped
Garlic = 2 cloves, sliced
Tomatoes = 4, chopped
Mustard, Dijon (or yellow) = small amount
Vinegar = Any type, preferably Balsamic, 1 teaspoon
Cilantro or Basil or Mint leaves

Optional:
Sea- Salt = 1 teaspoon
Cumin seeds (or powder) or Caraway seeds = 1/2 teaspoon
Turmeric powder = 1/2 teaspoon
Black pepper = 1 teaspoon OR Cayenne pepper = 1/2 teaspoon

Add olive oil onion, garlic and celery in a big pot and place it on low heat. Cook for about 5 minutes, stirring frequently, until the onions have turned yellowish brown.

Then add chicken chunks, mustard and tomatoes. Turn the heat to medium and cook for about 5 minutes, stirring frequently. Turn heat to low. Add bell pepper. Cook uncovered for about 3 -5 minutes. Add cilantro, basil or mint leaves.

Optional:
In the beginning, add salt, turmeric powder, cumin (or caraway seeds), black pepper OR cayenne pepper.

Ground Turkey or Ground Chicken - Bell Pepper

Cooking Time = About 25 minutes

Ingredients:

Ground turkey (or chicken) = 1 pound
Bell pepper = 2 medium, any color, preferably red, cut into chunks
Olive oil = 2 tablespoons
Onion = 1 medium, chopped
Garlic = 2 or 3 cloves, sliced
Tomatoes = 2 medium, chopped
Sea-Salt = ½ teaspoon (to taste)
Turmeric powder = ¼ teaspoon
Basil leaves, preferably fresh = 8-10 OR 1 teaspoon dried

Optional:

Cumin (or Caraway seeds) = 1/2 teaspoon
Cayenne pepper or black pepper = 1/2 teaspoon

Use a medium size pot. Sauté onion and garlic in olive oil until translucent. Add 1/4 cup of water, turmeric powder and tomatoes, and cover. Cook for another 5 minutes on low heat.

Then, add ground turkey or chicken. Break up meat so that it is in small pieces. Cook until pink is gone, which takes about 5 - 10 minutes.

Add bell pepper. Cook on low heat, uncovered, for about 3 -5 minutes. Add basil leaves in the end.

Optional:
In the beginning, add cumin (or caraway seeds), black pepper OR cayenne pepper after adding water.

Ground Turkey or Ground Chicken - Zucchini

Cooking Time = About 25 minutes

Ingredients:

Ground turkey (or chicken) = 1 pound
Zucchini = 2 medium, unpeeled, sliced
Olive oil = 2 tablespoons
Onion = 1 medium, chopped
Garlic = 2 or 3 cloves, sliced
Tomatoes = 2 medium, chopped
Clove powder = 1/2 teaspoon
Sea-Salt = ½ teaspoon (to taste)
Turmeric = ¼ teaspoon
Basil OR Oregano leaves = Fresh, 8-10 OR dried = 1 teaspoon

Optional:

Cumin (or Caraway seeds) = 1/2 teaspoon
Cayenne pepper or black pepper = 1/2 teaspoon

Use a medium size pot. Sauté onion and garlic in olive oil until translucent. Add 1/4 cup of water, turmeric powder and tomatoes, and cover. Cook for another 5 minutes on low heat.

Then, add ground turkey or chicken. Break up meat so that it is in small pieces. Cook until pink is gone, which takes about 5 - 10 minutes.

Add zucchini and cloves. Cook on low heat, uncovered, for about 3 -5 minutes. Add oregano or basil leaves.

Optional:
In the beginning, add cumin (or caraway seeds), black pepper OR cayenne pepper after adding water.

Ground Turkey or Ground Chicken - Green Beans

Cooking Time = About 25 minutes

Ingredients:

Ground turkey (or chicken) = 1 pound
Green beans = 20
Olive oil = 2 tablespoons
Onion = 1 medium, chopped
Garlic = 2 or 3 cloves, sliced
Tomatoes = 2 medium, chopped
Dijon mustard = 1 tablespoon
Sea-Salt = ½ teaspoon (to taste)
Turmeric = ¼ teaspoon
Cilantro, Basil or Oregano leaves = fresh 8-10 or dried, 1 teaspoon

Optional:

Cumin (or Caraway seeds) = 1/2 teaspoon
Cayenne pepper or black pepper = 1/2 teaspoon

Use a medium size pot. Sauté onion and garlic in olive oil until translucent. Add 1/4 cup of water, turmeric powder and tomatoes, and cover. Cook for another 5 minutes on low heat.

Then, add ground turkey or chicken. Break up meat so that it is in small pieces. Cook until pink is gone, which takes about 5 - 10 minutes. Add green beans and Dijon mustard. Cook on low heat, uncovered, for about 5 - 10 minutes. In the end, add cilantro or oregano or basil leaves.

Optional:
In the beginning, add cumin (or caraway seeds), black pepper OR cayenne pepper after adding water.

Ground Turkey or Ground Chicken - Eggplant

Cooking Time = About 25 minutes

Ingredients:

Ground turkey (or chicken) = 1 pound
Eggplant = 2, preferably Japanese or Chinese, sliced
Yogurt = 2 tablespoons
Olive oil = 2 tablespoons
Onion = 1 medium, chopped
Garlic = 2 or 3 cloves, sliced
Tomatoes = 2 medium, chopped
Sea-Salt = ½ teaspoon (to taste)
Turmeric = ¼ teaspoon
Basil leaves = Preferably fresh 8-10 or dried, 1 teaspoon
Pine nuts = a handful

Optional:

Cumin (or Caraway seeds) = 1/2 teaspoon
Cayenne pepper or black pepper = 1/2 teaspoon

Use a medium size pot. Sauté onion and garlic in olive oil until translucent. Add 1/4 cup of water, turmeric powder and tomatoes, and cover. Cook for another 5 minutes on low heat.

Then, add ground turkey or chicken. Break up meat so that it is in small pieces. Cook until pink is gone, which takes about 5 - 10 minutes. Add eggplant and yogurt. Cook on low heat, covered, for about 10 minutes. In the end, add pine nuts and basil leaves.

Optional:
In the beginning, add cumin (or caraway seeds), black pepper OR cayenne pepper after adding water.

Ground Turkey or Ground Chicken - Spinach

Cooking Time = About 25 minutes

Ingredients:

Ground turkey (or chicken) = 1 pound
Spinach = 4-5 handfuls
Yogurt = 2 tablespoons
Olive oil = 2 tablespoons
Onion = 1 medium, chopped
Garlic = 2 or 3 cloves, sliced
Tomatoes = 2 medium, sliced
Sea-Salt = ½ teaspoon (to taste)
Turmeric = ¼ teaspoon
Cilantro or oregano leaves = Preferably fresh 8-10 OR dried, teaspoon dried

Optional:

Cumin (or Caraway seeds) = 1/2 teaspoon
Cayenne pepper or black pepper = 1/2 teaspoon

Use a medium size pot. Sauté onion and garlic in olive oil until translucent. Add 1/4 cup of water, turmeric powder and tomatoes, and cover. Cook for another 5 minutes on low heat.

Then, add ground turkey or chicken. Break up meat so that it is in small pieces. Cook until pink is gone, which takes about 5 - 10 minutes. Add spinach and yogurt. Cook on low heat, uncovered, for about 10 minutes. In the end, add cilantro or oregano leaves.

Optional:
In the beginning, add cumin (or caraway seeds), black pepper OR cayenne pepper after adding water.

Ground Turkey or Ground Chicken - Carrots

Cooking Time = About 25 minutes

Ingredients:

Ground turkey (or chicken) = 1 pound
Carrots= 3 medium sized, peeled, chopped
Celery = 1 stick, chopped
Olive oil = 2 tablespoons
Onion = 1 medium, chopped
Garlic = 2 or 3 cloves, sliced
Tomatoes = 2 medium , sliced
Sea-Salt = ½ teaspoon (to taste)
Cinnamon = ¼ teaspoon
Basil leaves = Preferably fresh or 1 teaspoon dried

Optional:

Cumin (or Caraway seeds) = 1/2 teaspoon
Cayenne pepper or black pepper = 1/2 teaspoon

Use a medium size pot. Sauté onion and garlic in olive oil until translucent. Add 1/4 cup of water, celery and tomatoes, and cover. Cook for another 5 minutes on low heat.

Then, add ground turkey or chicken. Break up meat so that it is in small pieces. Cook until pink is gone, which takes about 5 - 10 minutes. Add carrots. Cook on low heat, uncovered, for about 3 -5 minutes. In the end, add basil leaves.

Optional:
In the beginning, add cumin (or caraway seeds), black pepper OR cayenne pepper after adding water.

Ground Turkey or Ground Chicken - Sweet Peas

Cooking Time = About 25 minutes

Ingredients:

Ground turkey (or chicken) = 1 pound
Sweet peas = 1 cup
Olive oil = 2 tablespoons
Onion = 1 medium, chopped
Garlic = 2 or 3 cloves, sliced
Tomatoes = 2 , sliced
Sea-Salt = ½ teaspoon (to taste)
Turmeric = ¼ teaspoon
Basil and Oregano leaves = Preferably fresh 8-10 or dried, 1 teaspoon

Optional:

Cumin (or Caraway seeds) = 1/2 teaspoon
Cayenne pepper or black pepper = 1/2 teaspoon

Use a medium size pot. Sauté onion and garlic in olive oil until translucent. Add 1/4 cup of water, turmeric powder and tomatoes, and cover. Cook for another 5 minutes on low heat.

Then, add ground turkey or chicken. Break up meat so that it is in small pieces. Cook until pink is gone, which takes about 5 - 10 minutes. Add sweet peas. Cook on low heat, uncovered, for about 3 - 5 minutes. In the end, add basil and oregano leaves.

Optional:
In the beginning, add cumin (or caraway seeds), black pepper OR cayenne pepper after adding water.

Ground Turkey or Ground Chicken - Cauliflower

Cooking Time = About 25 minutes

Ingredients:

Ground turkey (or chicken) = 1 pound
Cauliflower = 1 cauliflower head, chopped into 10 -12 small pieces
Ginger root = A piece about 2 inches x 1 inch. Peeled and sliced
Yogurt = 2 tablespoons
Celery = 1 stick, chopped
Olive oil = 2 tablespoons
Onion = 1 medium, chopped
Garlic = 2 or 3 cloves, sliced
Tomatoes = 2 , sliced
Sea-Salt = ½ teaspoon (to taste)
Turmeric = ¼ teaspoon
Cilantro or Basil or Mint leaves = Preferably fresh 8-10 or dried, 1 teaspoon

Optional:

Cumin (or Caraway seeds) = 1/2 teaspoon
Cayenne pepper or black pepper = 1/2 teaspoon

Use a medium size pot. Sauté onion and garlic in olive oil until translucent. Add 1/4 cup of water, turmeric powder, ginger, celery and tomatoes, and cover. Cook for another 5 minutes on low heat.

Then, add ground turkey or chicken. Break up meat so that it is in small pieces. Cook until pink is gone, which takes about 5 - 10 minutes. Add cauliflower and yogurt. Cook on low heat, covered, for about 15 minutes, stirring sparingly. In the end, add cilantro or basil or mint leaves.

Optional:
In the beginning, add cumin (or caraway seeds), black pepper OR cayenne pepper after adding water.

Beef or Lamb - Cauliflower - Bell Pepper

Cooking Time = About 35 minutes

Ingredients:

Beef or Lamb for Stew = 1 Lbs., cut into chunks
Cauliflower = 1 of the whole cauliflower head, chopped into 10 -12 small pieces
Bell pepper = 2 medium, any color, preferably red, cut into chunks
Yogurt = 2 tablespoons
Olive oil = 6 tablespoons
Celery = 1 stalk, sliced into small pieces
Onion = 1 medium, chopped
Garlic = 2 clove, sliced
Ginger root = A piece about 2 inches x 1 inch. Peeled and sliced
Mustard, Dijon, (or regular, yellow) = small amount
Vinegar = Any type, preferably Balsamic, 1 teaspoon
Sea-Salt = 1 teaspoon
Cumin seeds (or powder) or Caraway seeds = 1/2 teaspoon
Turmeric powder = 1/2 teaspoon
Cilantro OR Basil Or Mint leaves = Fresh 8-10 OR dried, 1 teaspoon

Optional:

Black pepper = 1 teaspoon OR Cayenne pepper = 1/2 teaspoon

In a big pot on low heat, add olive oil and warm. Add onion, ginger, cumin seeds and salt. Cook for about 5 minutes, stirring frequently, until the onions have turned yellowish brown. Add beef chunks, mustard, turmeric powder, vinegar and yogurt.

Optional: Add black pepper OR cayenne pepper.

Turn the heat to medium and cook for about 5 minutes, stirring frequently.

Turn heat to low. Add cauliflower, tomatoes, garlic and celery. Cover and let it cook for about 30 minutes. Check only once or twice to make sure water is still there. Avoid frequent uncovering. It will reduce the amount of steam, which is cooking the beef and cauliflower.

Uncover. Add bell pepper. Cook uncovered for about 5 minutes. Cook longer to dry it up, if you wish. In the end, add cilantro or mint or basil leaves. Mix well.

Beef or Lamb - Spinach

Cooking Time = About 45 minutes

Ingredients:

Beef or Lamb for Stew = 1 Lbs., cut into chunks
Spinach = about 4 handfuls
Yogurt = 2 tablespoons
Olive oil = 8-10 tablespoons
Butter = 1/2 stick
Celery = 1 stalk, chopped
Onion = 2, medium, chopped
Garlic = 2 clove, sliced
Ginger root = A piece about 2 inches x 1 inch. Peeled and sliced
Mustard = Dijon or regular yellow, small amount
Vinegar = Any type, preferably Balsamic, 1 teaspoon
Sea-Salt = 1 teaspoon
Turmeric powder = 1/2 teaspoon
Cilantro or Basil or Mint leaves = 8-10 fresh OR dried, 1 teaspoon

Optional:

Mustard greens = 4 handfuls, chopped
Collard greens = 2 handfuls
Black pepper = 1 teaspoon OR Cayenne pepper = 1/2 teaspoon.

In a medium size pot on low heat, add 4 tablespoons of olive oil, one chopped onion, ginger and salt. Cook for about 5 minutes, stirring frequently until the onions have turned yellowish brown. Add beef or lamb chunks, mustard, turmeric powder, vinegar and yogurt.

Optional: Add black pepper, OR cayenne pepper.

Turn the heat to medium and cook for about 5 minutes, stirring frequently.

In a separate large pot, add 4 - 6 tablespoons of olive oil, garlic, one chopped onion and spinach.

Optional: Add mustard greens and collard greens.

Cover and let it cook for about 30 minutes. Then, pour it into a blender and grind on low until all leaves are well ground. Pour it back into the large pot.

Empty beef or lamb chunks mixture into this large pot. Mix well. Add butter. Cook for another 15 - 20 minutes on low heat, uncovered, till it is not runny any more.

In the end, add cilantro or mint or basil leaves. Mix well.

Juicy Steak

Ingredients:

Steak = Two approx. 12 ounce New York or Filet Mignon cuts
Yogurt = 3 tablespoons
Olive oil = 6 tablespoons
Bell pepper = 1/2, preferable red, chopped
Vinegar = 1 tablespoon
Mustard, Dijon = 2 tablespoons
Garlic powder = 1 tablespoon
Garlic, fresh = 1 clove, peeled and sliced
Lime (or Lemon) = 1, halved
Sea-Salt = 1 teaspoon
Onion = 1 small, chopped
Tomatoes = 2 medium, chopped
Basil leaves, fresh = 1 cup
Black olives = 10, halved
Capers = 2 tablespoons
Mushrooms = 4-5 white mushrooms, sliced
Cranberries = a handful

Optional:

Pine nuts = a handful
Black Pepper = 1 teaspoon or Cayenne pepper = 1/2 teaspoon

Step 1

Marinate steaks in a pan: Add 1 tablespoon olive oil, 1 tablespoon yogurt, 1 tablespoon Dijon mustard, vinegar, garlic powder and 1 teaspoon of salt. Squeeze and add lime (or lemon).

Optional: Add black pepper or cayenne pepper. Mix well.

Place Steaks in this marinate mixture. Cover well with the marinate mixture by flipping them over several times. Let sit for about 30 - 60 minutes.

Step 2

Make your own <u>pesto</u>: Add basil leaves, 2 tablespoons of water, 2 tablespoons of olive oil, red bell pepper, 1 teaspoon of salt and garlic powder into a blender.

<u>Optional</u>: Add a handful of pine nuts.

Turn the blender on for a minute or so, until the basil leaves are ground into a paste. Empty your pesto into a container.

Step 3

Make your own <u>sauce</u>: In a small pan on low heat, add 3 tablespoons olive oil, onions and sliced garlic. Cook for about 5 minutes. Stir frequently. Onions should be translucent, yellowish but not brown. Then, add 1/2 cup water, 2 tablespoons yogurt, 1 tablespoon Dijon mustard, tomatoes and 1 tablespoon homemade pesto. Mix well. Cook on low heat for another 25-30 minutes, stirring frequently, until it is paste like. In the end, add cranberries, capers, black olives and mushrooms. Your own sauce is now ready.

Step 4

Broil steaks in an Oven for about 5-10 minutes each side, depending upon your taste of rare, medium or well done.

Step 5

Transfer steaks onto a dish. Cover them with your already cooked sauce. Let sit for about 5 minutes before serving.

Tip: Serve it with Salad No. 2 or 3. Great for lunch or dinner.

Zesty Lamb Chops

Ingredients:

Lamb chops = 8
Yogurt = 4 tablespoons
Olive oil = 2 tablespoons
Garlic powder = 1 teaspoon
Ginger powder= 1 teaspoon
Cumin Powder = 1/2 teaspoon
Coriander powder = 1/2 teaspoon
Clove powder = 1/2 teaspoon
Basil dried leaves = 1 teaspoon
Oregano dried leaves = 1 teaspoon
Mustard, Dijon or regular yellow = small amount
Apple cider vinegar = 1 teaspoon

Optional:

Black pepper = 1 teaspoon OR Cayenne pepper = 1/2 teaspoon

In a large pan, add olive oil, yogurt, ginger, garlic, cumin, coriander, clove powder, basil leaves, oregano leaves, Dijon mustard and vinegar. Add a couple of tablespoons of water. Mix well to form a paste.

Optional: Add black pepper OR cayenne pepper.

Place lamb chops in the pan. Holding them by their bony stick, cover them well with the paste on each side. Cover them and marinate for 1 - 2 hours.

Place the pan on a stove, uncovered, at medium to high heat for 5 minutes. Then, lower the heat and cook for another 5-10 minutes, depending upon your taste - rare, medium or well done.

Tip: Use a side dish of one of the salads in this book.

Zesty Lamb Chops - Broccoli - Cauliflower - Eggplant

Ingredients:

Lamb chops, cooked according to the previous recipe
Broccoli = 4 - 6 florets
Cauliflower = 4 - 6 florets
Eggplant = 2, preferably Japanese or Chinese, sliced
Olive oil = 2 tablespoons
Onion = 1 medium, chopped
Mustard, Dijon = 1 tablespoon
Tomatoes = 2, chopped
Cumin seeds = 1/2 teaspoon
Turmeric = ¼ teaspoon

Optional:

Cayenne pepper or black pepper = 1/2 teaspoon.

In a large pan, add olive oil and 1/2 cup of water. Add broccoli, cauliflower, eggplant, cumin seeds, turmeric and Dijon mustard.

Optional: Add black pepper OR cayenne pepper.

Cover and cook on medium heat. Let it cook for about 10 minutes. Check only once or twice to make sure water is still there. Avoid frequent uncovering. It will reduce the amount of steam, which is cooking the vegetables.

Add onions and tomatoes. Turn the heat to low and cook for about 5 minutes, stirring frequently. In the end, add pre-cooked lamb chops. Cover and let it cook on low heat for 2- 3 minutes.

Zesty Beef Stir Fry

Cooking time = About 15 minutes

Ingredients:

Beef for stir fry = 1/2 to 3/4 Lbs., cut into chunks
Yogurt = 2 Tablespoons
Celery = 1 stalk, sliced into small pieces
Zucchini = 1, medium, peeled and sliced
Carrot = 2, small, peeled and cut into small pieces
Bell Pepper = 1, medium, cut into small pieces
Tomato = 1, medium, chopped
Basil leaves = 5, fresh or 1/2 teaspoonful of dried, crushed leaves
Onion = 1, medium, chopped
Ginger = Fresh, 1 inch X 2 inches, peeled and sliced or 1/2 teaspoon of powdered ginger
Garlic = 1 clove, peeled and sliced
Mustard, yellow = 1/2 tablespoon
Sea-Salt = 1/2 teaspoon
Balsamic vinegar = 1/4 teaspoon
Olive Oil = 2 Tablespoon

Optional:

Yogurt = 2 tablespoons
Cayenne pepper or black pepper = 1/2 teaspoon
Turmeric = ¼ teaspoon
Coriander, ground = 1 teaspoon
Cumin, powder = 1 teaspoon
Cloves, whole = 5

In a medium hot wok, add olive oil, onion, celery, zucchini and yogurt. After a couple of minutes, add beef. Stir continuously. After a couple of minutes, add salt, garlic, ginger, vinegar and mustard.

Optional: Add coriander, cumin, turmeric, cloves and hot cayenne pepper. Continue to stir.

After about 5 minutes, add 1/2 cup of water. Add carrots and cover. Lower the heat and let it cook for another 5 minutes. Stir periodically.

Then, add bell pepper, tomato and basil leaves. Cook for another 2-3 minutes. Let it cool for a few minutes before serving.

Ground Beef - Sweet Peas - Carrots - Olives

Cooking time = About 25 minutes

Ingredients:

Ground beef = 1 pound
Sweet Peas = 1 cup
Carrots = 3 medium sized, peeled, chopped
Mustard, Dijon = 1/2 tablespoon
Black olives = 15, halved
Celery = 1 stick, chopped
Ginger root = A piece about 2 inches x 1 inch. Peeled and sliced
Olive oil = 3 tablespoons
Onion = 1 medium, chopped
Garlic = 2 or 3 cloves, sliced
Sea-Salt = ½ teaspoon (to taste)
Cilantro or Basil leaves = Preferably fresh 8-10 OR dried, 1 teaspoon
Yogurt = 2 tablespoons

Optional:

Cayenne pepper or black pepper = 1/2 teaspoon
Turmeric = ¼ teaspoon
Coriander, ground = 1 teaspoon
Cumin, powder = 1 teaspoon

Add olive oil, onions, celery, ginger, and garlic in a medium size pot. Cook on medium heat for about 5-10 minutes, until onions are translucent and yellowish. Stir frequently.

Add ground beef. Break up meat so that it is in small pieces. Cook until pink is gone, which takes about 5 minutes. Add yogurt and Dijon mustard and cook for a couple of minutes. Lower the heat, and add sweet peas and carrots.

Optional: Add cayenne pepper or black pepper, turmeric, coriander and cumin at the beginning.

Cook on low heat, uncovered, for about 10 -15 minutes, stirring frequently. In the end, add black olives, cilantro or basil leaves.

Tip: You can make lettuce wraps out of it.

Beef Stew 1

Cooking time = About 100 minutes

Ingredients:

Beef stew meat = 1 pound, cut into chunks
Yogurt, plain = 3 tablespoons
Carrots = 2, medium, peeled and cut into pieces
Turnip = 1, peeled, chopped into small pieces
Celery = 1 stalk, cut into small pieces
Onion = 1 medium, peeled, cut into chunks
Garlic = 2 cloves, peeled, cut into small pieces
Ginger root = 1 small piece about 2 inches x 1 inch, peeled and cut into small pieces
Turmeric powder = 1/4 teaspoon
Coriander powder = 1/4 teaspoon
Cumin powder = 1/4 teaspoon
Paprika = 1/4 teaspoon
Sea-Salt = 1/2 teaspoon.
Balsamic vinegar = 1/4 teaspoon

Rinse Beef stew meat chunks and place them in a large pot. Add Yogurt, Onion, Celery, Turnip, Garlic, Ginger, Turmeric, Coriander, Cumin, Paprika, Salt and about 3 tablespoons of water. Mix well and marinate for about 5 minutes.

Then, cook on high heat. Stir frequently until the meat turns brown, about 5 minutes.

Add 3 cups of hot water. Cover and turn heat to very Low. Let cook for about 30 minutes, stirring periodically.

Add Carrots and let it simmer, covered, for another 60 minutes, stirring occasionally. Then, add Balsamic Vinegar. Stir and let it cool for about 5 minutes before serving.

Beef Stew 2

Cooking time = About 45 minutes

Ingredients:

Beef chunks = 1 - 2 Lbs., cut into chunks
Bell pepper = 1 - 2, cut into chunks
Spinach = 1 bunch (approximately 2 cups), washed
Celery Stick = 2, cut into small pieces
Tomatoes = 4 - 6 medium, cut into chunks
Yogurt, plain = 4 tablespoons
Cloves, whole = 4
Olive oil = 2 tablespoons
Turmeric = 1/2 teaspoon
Sea-Salt = 1/2 teaspoon
Cinnamon = 1 stick
Cumin seeds (or powder) = 1 teaspoon
Coriander ground = 1 teaspoon
Garlic = 2 cloves, sliced
Onions = 2 medium size, chopped
Ginger root, fresh = about 1/2 inch square, chopped

Optional:

Cayenne pepper = 1/2 to 1 teaspoon per your taste
Paprika = 1 to 2 teaspoons per your taste

In a large pot, add about 2-3 tablespoons of water, olive oil, onions, celery, salt, garlic, ginger, turmeric, cinnamon stick, cloves, cumin seeds and coriander powder and turn on heat to medium. Keep stirring frequently.

Optional:
Add Cayenne pepper OR paprika.

After about 5 minutes, add beef and yogurt. Mix in well. Adjust the heat to low and cover. Let it cook for about 30 minutes, stirring frequently.

Then, add spinach and bell pepper. Cover and let it cook for another 10 minutes, stirring frequently.

Add tomatoes, cover and let it cook another 5 minutes, stirring frequently.

* You can use Cayenne pepper if you like it hot OR Paprika which is very mild. You can also add two whole dried cayenne peppers if you like it extra hot.

FISH

White Fish - Pan Fried

Cooking Time = About 15 minutes

Ingredients:

White Fish (Fresh water) filet = 2 (about 2/3 Lbs.)
Olive oil = 1 tablespoon
Vinegar = 1/2 teaspoon
Mustard, yellow or Dijon = small amount
Lime (or lemon) = 1, cut in half
Garlic powder = 1 teaspoon
Sea-Salt = 1/2 teaspoon
Basil leaves and Rosemary leaves = a few, preferably fresh

Optional:

Black Pepper = 1 teaspoon OR Cayenne pepper = 1/2 teaspoon

First marinate fish filet: Put olive oil into a large pan. Place fish filets in it, side by side. Squeeze lime (or lemon) on the filets. Then, sprinkle garlic powder.

Optional: Add black pepper OR cayenne pepper.

Then, squeeze mustard directly on the filet. Let it sit for about 5 minutes.

Cook the filets in a pan on medium heat for about 5 minutes. Then, turn the filets over and cook for another 5 minutes or so, depending on the thickness of the filets.

Turn heat off. Sprinkle basil leaves and fresh rosemary leaves over filets.

Trout - Pan Fried

Cooking Time = About 20 minutes

Ingredients:

Trout filets = 2 (about 2/3 Lbs.)
Olive oil = 6 tablespoons
Vinegar = 1 tablespoon
Mustard, Dijon = 1 tablespoon
Garlic powder = 1 tablespoon
Lime (or lemon) = 1, cut in half
Sea-Salt = 1/2 teaspoon
Onion = 1 small, chopped
Tomatoes, cherry = 8-10, halved
Basil leaves, fresh = 1 cup
Garlic, fresh = 1 clove, peeled and sliced
Black olives = 10
Capers = 2 tablespoons

Optional:

Black Pepper = 1 teaspoon OR Cayenne pepper = 1/2 teaspoon

Step 1:

Start out by making your own pesto as follows: Add a cupful of fresh basil leaves, 2 tablespoons of water, 2 tablespoons olive oil, black olives, and fresh garlic slices into a blender. Turn it on for a minute or so, until the basil leaves are ground into a paste. Empty your pesto into a container.

Step 2:

Marinate fish filet: Put one tablespoon of olive oil into a large pan. Add Dijon mustard, vinegar, garlic powder and salt, and squeeze lime (or lemon).

Optional: Add black pepper or cayenne pepper. Mix well.

Place fish filets in this mixture. Cover them well with the marinate mixture, by flipping them over several times. Let them marinate for about 5 minutes.

Step 3:

Make your own <u>sauce</u>: In a small pan, add 3 tablespoons of olive oil, onions and tomatoes, and cook on low heat for about 5 minutes. Stir frequently. You want onions to turn translucent, yellowish but not brown. Then, add one tablespoon of your own pesto. Mix well. Let it cook for another couple of minutes, stirring frequently.

Step 4:

Place fish pan on the stove at medium heat and cook for about 1-2 minutes. Then, turn the filets over and cook for another 1-2 minutes. Turn filets over again and cook for 1-2 minutes. Flip and cook for another 1-2 minutes. Total fish cooking time about 6 minutes.

Step 5:

Transfer fish filets onto a dish. Cover them with your already cooked sauce. Let sit for a couple of minutes before serving.

Tip: Serve it with Salad No. 2 or 3. Great for light dinner.

Salmon - Pan Fried

Cooking Time = About 20 minutes

Ingredients:

Salmon filets (farm-raised) = 2 (about 2/3 Lbs.)
Yogurt = 2 tablespoons
Olive oil = 6 tablespoons
Bell pepper = 1/2, preferable red, chopped
Vinegar = 1 tablespoon
Mustard, Dijon = 2 tablespoons
Garlic powder = 2 tablespoons
Garlic, fresh = 1 clove, peeled and sliced
Lime (or lemon) = 1, halved
Sea-Salt = 1 teaspoon
Onion = 1 small, chopped
Tomatoes, cherry = 8-10, halved
Basil leaves, fresh = 1 cup
Black olives = 10, halved
Capers = 2 tablespoons

Optional:

Cranberries = a handful
Pine nuts = a handful
Black Pepper = 1 teaspoon or Cayenne pepper = 1/2 teaspoon

Step 1:

Start out by making your own pesto: Add 1 cup of fresh basil leaves, 2 tablespoons water, 2 tablespoons olive oil, red bell pepper, 1/2 teaspoon of salt and 1 tablespoon of garlic powder into a blender. Optional: Add a handful of pine nuts. Turn the blender on for a minute or so, until the basil leaves are ground into a paste. Empty your pesto into a container.

Step 2:

Marinate fish filet in a pan: Add 1 tablespoon olive oil, 1 tablespoon Dijon mustard, 1 tablespoon vinegar, 1 tablespoon garlic powder and 1/2 teaspoon salt. Squeeze and add lime (or lemon).

Optional: Add black pepper or cayenne pepper. Mix well.

Place fish filets in this marinate mixture and cover them well with the marinate mixture by flipping them over several times. Let sit for about 5 minutes.

Step 3:

Make your own sauce: In a small pan on low heat, add 3 tablespoons olive oil, onions and sliced garlic. Cook for about 5 minutes. Stir frequently. Onions should be translucent, yellowish but not brown. Then, add 1/2 cup of water, yogurt, 1 tablespoon Dijon mustard, tomatoes and your own pesto. Mix well. Let cook on low heat for another 25-30 minutes, stirring frequently, until it is paste like. In the end, add capers and black olives. Your own sauce is now ready.

Step 4:

Cook fish in marinating pan at medium heat for about 2-3 minutes. Then, turn the filets over and cook for another 2 -3 minutes. Turn filets over again and cook for 1-2 minutes each side, one more time. Total fish cooking time about 10 minutes.

Step 5:

Transfer fish filets to a dish. Cover them with your already cooked sauce. Let it sit for a couple of minutes before serving.

Tip: Serve it with Salad No. 2 or 3. Great for light dinner.

ACKNOWLEDGEMENTS

I gratefully acknowledge Georgie Huntington Zaidi, my editor, who did an extraordinary job of transforming this complex medical book into an easy read. On a personal note, I appreciate her every day for being my soul-mate.

I am deeply grateful to my wonderful patients who graciously granted me permission to include their case studies without which the book would have been *colorless*. I also sincerely acknowledge the brilliant scientific work of many researchers devoted to the field of Thyroid.

Sarfraz Zaidi, M.D.

www.DoctorZaidi.com

About Dr. Zaidi

Dr. Sarfraz Zaidi is a leading Endocrinologist in the U.S.A. He is a medical expert on Thyroid, Diabetes, Vitamin D and Stress Management. He is the director of the Jamila Diabetes and Endocrine Medical Center in Thousand Oaks, California. He is a former assistant Clinical Professor of Medicine at UCLA.

Books and Articles

Dr. Zaidi is the author of these books: **"Stress Cure Now"**, **"Hypothyroidism And Hashimoto's Thyroiditis"**, **"Power of Vitamin D"**, **"Take Charge of Your Diabetes,"** and **"Stress Management For Teenagers, Parents And Teachers."** In addition, he has authored numerous articles in prestigious medical journals.

Memberships

Dr. Zaidi is a Member of the American Association of Clinical Endocrinologists (AACE). In 1997, Dr. Zaidi was inducted as a Fellow to the American College of Physicians (FACP). In 1999, he was honored to be a Fellow of the American College of Endocrinology (FACE).

Speaker

Dr. Zaidi has been a guest speaker at medical conferences and also frequently gives lectures to the public. He has been interviewed on TV, newspapers and national magazines. Dr. Zaidi is the former director of the Endocrine Clinic at the Olive-View UCLA Medical Center where he taught resident physicians undergoing training in Diabetes and Endocrinology.

Internet

Dr. Zaidi also regularly writes on websites including:

www.OnlineMedinfo.com which provides in-depth knowledge about endocrine disorders such as Thyroid, Vitamin D, Parathyroid,

Osteoporosis, Obesity, PreDiabetes, Metabolic Syndrome, Menopause, Low Testosterone, Adrenal, Pituitary and more.

www.DiabetesSpecialist.com which is dedicated to providing extensive knowledge to Diabetics.

www.InnerPeaceAndLove.com which is an inspirational website exploring the Mind-Body connection.

He regularly writes on his Blog.
www.onlinemedinfo.com/blog/

He has done educational YouTube videos about Vitamin D at www.youtube.com/user/georgie6988
And about Insulin resistance, diabetes and heart disease at www.youtube.com/user/TheDiabetesEducation

His main website: **www.DoctorZaidi.com**

Other Books by Dr. Sarfraz Zaidi

"Hypothyroidism And Hashimoto's Thyroiditis"

The current treatment of Hypothyroidism is superficial and unsatisfactory. Patients continue to suffer from the symptoms of Hypothyroidism, despite taking thyroid pills. Even worse, there is no treatment for Hashimoto's Thyroiditis, the root cause of hypothyroidism in a large number of patients.
Dr. Zaidi has made a breakthrough discovery about the real cause of Hashimoto's Thyroiditis, and how to effectively treat it. He has also made new insights into the causes of Hypothyroidism. Based on these ground-breaking discoveries, he has developed a revolutionary approach to treat Hypothyroidism and cure Hashimoto's Thyroiditis. In "Hypothyroidism And Hashimoto's Thyroiditis, A Breakthrough Approach to Effective Treatment," you will find out.

- Why you continue to suffer from symptoms of Hypothyroidism, despite taking thyroid pills?
- What really is Hypothyroidism?
- What are the symptoms of Hypothyroidism?
- Why the diagnosis of Hypothyroidism is often missed?
- Why the current treatment approach of hypothyroidism is unscientific?
- Why the usual tests for thyroid function are inaccurate and misleading?
- What actually causes Hypothyroidism?
- What is the root cause of Hashimoto's Thyroiditis, besides genetics?
- What other conditions are commonly associated with Hashimoto's Thyroiditis?
- How to effectively treat Hypothyroidism?
- How to cure Hashimoto's Thyroiditis?
- And a detailed thyroid diet that works.

"Stress Management For Teenagers, Parents And Teachers"

Using the blazing torch of logic, Dr. Zaidi cuts through the stress triangle of teenagers, parents and teachers. This original, profound and breakthrough approach is completely different from the usual, customary approaches to manage stress, which simply work as a band-aid, while the volcano underneath continues to smolder. Sooner or later, it erupts through the paper thin layers of these superficial strategies. Dr. Zaidi guides you step by step on how you can be free of various forms of stress. From peer pressure, to stress from education, to conflict between teenagers, parents and teachers, to anxiety, addictions and ADD, Dr. Zaidi covers every aspect of stress teenagers, parents and teachers experience in their day to day life. Dr. Zaidi's new approach ushers in a new era in psychology, yet this book is such an easy read. It's like talking to a close friend for practical, useful yet honest advice that works.

"Stress Cure Now"

In his ground breaking book, Dr. Zaidi describes a truly *New* approach to deal with stress. Dr. Zaidi's strategy to cure stress is based on his personal awakening, in-depth medical knowledge and vast clinical experience. It is simple, direct, original and therefore, profound. He uses logic - the common sense that every human is born with. Using the torch of logic, Dr. Zaidi shows you that the true root cause of stress actually resides inside you, not out there. Therefore, the solution must also resides inside you. In **"Stress Cure Now,"** Dr. Zaidi guides you to see the true root cause of your stress, in its deepest layers. Only then you can get rid of it from its roots, once and for all.

"Power of Vitamin D"

In this book, Dr. Zaidi provides compelling, comprehensive, yet very practical knowledge about vitamin D deficiency, its health consequences, its diagnosis and treatment (without the risk of toxicity). Dr. Zaidi illustrates important practical points by including real case studies from his clinical practice.

"Take Charge of Your Diabetes"

Insulin resistance is the root cause of diabetes in a majority of people, yet most have not even heard of it. In "Take Charge of Your Diabetes," Dr. Zaidi showcases his ground breaking *5-step strategy* to treat diabetes. Using this approach, learn how Dr. Zaidi's patients achieve excellent control of diabetes, prevent complications of diabetes and above all, do not end up on insulin shots. Learn how those who have been on insulin for years are able to come off insulin.

Dr. Zaidi's website
www.DoctorZaidi.com

VITAMIN D3

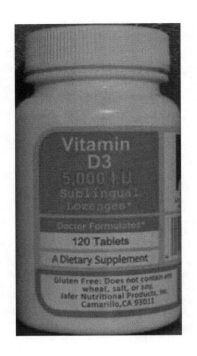

Jafer Nutritional Products, in collaboration with Dr. Sarfraz Zaidi, MD, now makes available a high quality Vitamin D3 formula for Sublingual absorption.

Each tablet contains **5000 IU** of Vitamin D3.

Call (805) 495-7143 or Visit www.DoctorZaidi.com

VITAMIN B12

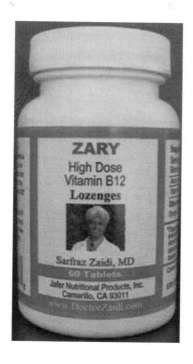

ZARY is a product of Jafer Nutritional Products, which is a vitamin manufacturer of the highest quality.

ZARY is created in collaboration with Dr. Sarfraz Zaidi, MD.

It contains Vitamin B12 in a high dose of 1000 mcg per tablet.

It is formulated as throat lozenges for sublingual absorption.

Call (805) 495-7143 or Visit www.DoctorZaidi.com

GLUPRIDE *Multi*

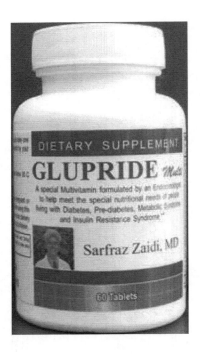

Glupride Multi is a unique vitamin/herbal formula

designed to promote health of people with

Diabetes, Pre-Diabetes and Metabolic Syndrome.

Glupride Multi is created by Sarfraz Zaidi, MD, a respected

Endocrinologist, an expert in the field of Diabetes and Insulin

Resistance Syndrome as well as author of the book,

"Take Charge Of Your Diabetes."

Call (805) 495-7143 or Visit www.DoctorZaidi.com

19126273R00147

Made in the USA
Middletown, DE
04 April 2015